What Do I Take?

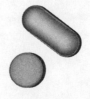

What Do I Take?
A Consumer's Guide to Nonprescription Drugs

Janice Fudyma

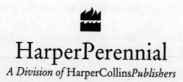

HarperPerennial
A Division of HarperCollins*Publishers*

HarperCollins books may be purchased for educational, business, or sales promotional use. For information, please write to: Special Markets Department, HarperCollins Publishers, Inc., 10 East 53rd Street, New York, New York 10022.

FIRST EDITION

LIBRARY OF CONGRESS CATALOG CARD NUMBER
ISBN 0-06-273422-9

Library of Congress Cataloging-in-Publication Data
Fudyma, Janice.
    What Do I Take? : a consumer's guide to non-prescription drugs / by Janice Fudyma.
        p. cm.
    ISBN 0-06-273422-9
    1. Drugs, Nonprescription—Popular works. 1. American Pharmaceutical Association.
    2. Title. 3. Title: An American Pharmaceutical Association guide
RM671.F83 1997
615'.1—dc21

97 98 99 00 RRD 10 9 8 7 6 5 4 3 2 1

To my daughters, Lauren and Kate, and my husband, Craig, whose common colds, allergies, and occasional bouts of the flu gave me the inspiration for this book. To my family, who shared their medical expertise, and especially to my brother John who helped make this book a reality. His guidance, time, and knowledge are greatly appreciated.

Table of Contents

The ailment listings, descriptions, symptoms, survey results, pharmacists' tips and advice on when to seek professional medical help.

continued on next page

* Children's products included.

continued on next page

* Children's products included.

General Warnings

Following are some key points that you should be aware of when taking over-the-counter medication. For specific warnings on each of the individual products refer to Section Two: About the Products.

Use all drugs only as directed. Do not exceed the recommended dosage.

If you are pregnant or nursing a baby, seek the advice of a health-care professional before taking any over-the-counter product.

Keep all drugs out of reach of children.

In case of accidental overdose or ingestion, call your doctor or contact a poison control center immediately. Prompt medical attention is critical for adults as well as children even if you do not notice any signs or symptoms.

If you are under a doctor's care for any medical condition **or are taking other drugs,** consult your pharmacist or doctor before taking any over-the-counter product.

If your symptoms persist or get worse, see a doctor promptly. If you experience symptoms that are unusual or unrelated to the condition for which you took the over-the-counter product, consult your doctor before taking any more.

Before taking an antihistamine you should know that this medication commonly causes drowsiness but can also cause excitability. If you have glaucoma, prostate disease, or breathing problems such as emphysema or chronic bronchitis, contact your pharmacist or doctor before taking any product containing an antihistamine.

Before taking a decongestant you should know that this medication may cause insomnia, anxiety, dizziness, and palpitations. If you have heart disease, high blood pressure, thyroid disease, diabetes, glaucoma, or prostate disease, contact your pharmacist or doctor before taking any product containing a decongestant.

Before taking an anti-inflammatory medication such as aspirin, ibuprofen, naproxen, etc., you should know that these medications may cause stomach upset. If you are allergic to aspirin, have asthma, stomach problems (such as heartburn, upset stomach, or stomach pain), peptic ulcers, or bleeding problems, contact your doctor before taking an over-the-counter anti-inflammatory medication. Do not give children any products containing aspirin, because of the risk of Reye's Syndrome, a rare but serious illness reported to be associated with aspirin.

If you have a history of allergy to local anesthetics, do not use products containing procaine, butacaine, benzocaine, or other "–caine" anesthetics.

Do not take two products that contain the same active ingredients.

Introduction

From the American Pharmaceutical Association

THE NATIONAL PROFESSIONAL SOCIETY OF PHARMACISTS

"What do I take?" indeed

Today more medications—and combinations of medications—are available without prescriptions than ever before. But just because a medication is sold "over the counter" doesn't mean it is harmless. Selecting the right nonprescription drug and taking it correctly is a serious matter. Here are some tips to help you make the best use of your nonprescription medicines.

Read the label carefully

For nonprescription medications, read the information on the label marked "Warnings" or "Drug Interaction Precautions." If the information is unclear, ask your pharmacist to clarify anything you don't understand.

Unless the label directs otherwise, store your nonprescription medicines at room temperature and away from moisture, heat, and direct light. Keep them securely closed in the original container and out of reach of children. The bathroom medicine cabinet is not recommended for storage, because humidity can decompose medications and alter their effect.

Use your pharmacist

Pharmacists are the health professionals with the most knowledge about medicines and their correct uses. Your pharmacist can advise you in selecting nonprescription medications for you and your family. Factors such as age, weight, symptoms, allergies, other medications you are taking, and other medical problems you have influence a medication's effectiveness. For example, a product that works for you may not be suitable for your children.

Choose a pharmacist...

- with whom you feel comfortable discussing health-related matters.
- who maintains complete records on the drugs you and your family members take.
- who will answer all your questions, counsel you, and monitor your response to medications.
- who will help you understand dosage instructions, potential side effects, and food and drug interactions.

When you find such a pharmacist, keep going back to that person to build a relationship, much as you would with a physician.

Your pharmacist can serve as your health-care advisor in stocking your home with important nonprescription medications and products. He or she can also advise you on possible cost savings. For example, nonprescription products bearing your local pharmacy's label are equivalent to national brand-name products and usually less expensive. Your pharmacist can answer your questions about alternative products.

Special Cautions

In some cases, two or more drugs taken together can change the way one or the other works in your body, possibly making them less safe or effective. These effects are known as drug interactions.

Give your pharmacist an up-to-date list of all the prescription and nonprescription medications and dietary supplements you take and the conditions for which you are taking them. The list should include the name of the product, the dosage, the prescribing physician (if applicable), and the date you started taking it. This list will help your pharmacist evaluate your medications for possible interactions.

Often certain foods and drinks and even certain activities should be avoided while taking a particular medication. Your pharmacist can tell you if a side effect is likely and how long the effect might last. Report to your pharmacist if any unexpected side effects occur.

Conclusion

Remember that, while you are in charge of making decisions about your health and self-care, your pharmacist is there to help. Ask your pharmacist how to make the best use of your medications.

JOHN A. GANS, PHARM. D.
Executive Vice President
American Pharmaceutical Association

About This Book

The Advisory Board

The pharmacists on the Advisory Board were recommended by the American Pharmaceutical Association (APhA) and represent both academia and community practice. These pharmacists helped to establish the final list of over-the-counter products for each ailment, determined the attributes by which each product would be rated and reviewed the pharmacists' tips in "Pharmacists Say..." and the section "About the Products."

The physician on the Advisory Board reviewed the ailment descriptions, symptoms, and "When to See the Doctor."

The Advisory Board consists of the following professionals who assisted me throughout the development of this book. I am grateful for their help and the time they dedicated.

The Products

The over-the-counter products for each ailment were chosen based on the following criteria:

- Each product had to be a nationally recognized name brand and not a generic or store brand version of the drug.

- Each product had to be sold and available nationally, not just sold by a particular store or in a particular region of the country.

- No recently released brand of over-the-counter product was included, because the pharmacists in the survey needed some experience with the products.

The products that were selected by the Advisory Board are by no means an endorsement.

The Survey

The survey was conducted by Burke Marketing Research, a division of Burke, Inc., of Cincinnati, Ohio. Burke is one of the nation's leading suppliers of custom survey research. In business for over 65 years, Burke Marketing Research works with companies to provide survey design, data collection, and analysis.

A random selection of all APhA members was chosen for participation in the survey. The pharmacists who participated were asked to rate each product on a 1 to 10 scale based on three of the following attributes: effectiveness, speed of relief, minimal side effects, ease of use, or desirable duration of relief, as well as to add any product that he or she thought should be included in the original list. Pharmacists were then requested to choose the one product they would most likely recommend. They were also asked to provide any comments on the products or recommendations that would be useful to the consumer. These comments and recommendations are included within each ailment under "Pharmacists Say...."

The 1 to 10 ratings in the product charts have been rounded to the nearest tenth of a point. The "Percentage of Pharmacists Who Most Often Recommend" scores have been rounded to the nearest whole number. Because of this rounding, the sum total may not always equal exactly 100 percent.

For a few products, there appears to be a discrepancy between their ranking in the "Percentage of Pharmacists Who Most Often Recommend" category and the scores they received in the various attribute categories. Certain products that received the highest scores for individual attributes may not have been the most often recommended, or vice versa.

There are a number of reasons why this situation can occur. For instance, the cost or palatability of a product—factors that were not considered in the individual attribute ratings—may have influenced a pharmacist to recommend one product over another. Or certain pharmacists may not be as likely to recommend a product if it is not well known by consumers in their area.

While these situations allow for, and may cause, a mismatch of rating and recommendation scores, their occurrence is insignificant.

The Survey Participants

Each pharmacist who participated in the survey is a community pharmacist with a minimum of three years of practice experience and is a current member of the American Pharmaceutical Association. Participants were also selected based on their geographic location in order to get national representation. After meeting these criteria, we then made a random selection of APhA pharmacists to participate in the project. The number of pharmacists we chose brought the final survey results to a 90 percent confidence level, plus or minus 8 percent.

How to Use This Book
'What Do I Take?' is divided into three sections.

SECTION ONE
Ailments

The ailments are listed alphabetically. (You can see an overview of these ailments in the Table of Contents.)

Each ailment is followed by a brief description and its symptoms.

The products selected by the Advisory Board to treat this ailment are listed alphabetically in the chart. EACH HAS BEEN RATED BY VARIOUS ATTRIBUTES BASED ON A 1 TO 10 SCALE, WITH 10 BEING THE HIGHEST SCORE. Pharmacists who participated in the survey were asked to choose the one product from the list they would recommend. The highest rating under each category is indicated in bold type.

'Pharmacists Say...' contains useful information from the pharmacists about the products or the ailment.

'See the Doctor...' appears at the end of each ailment and identifies when self-treatment needs to be stopped and professional medical evaluation initiated.

Dermatitis

Dermatitis is a term that encompasses a variety of ailments that cause an inflammation of the skin. One of the most common types, "contact dermatitis," is a result of touching a substance that causes a reaction, such as poison ivy or certain metals in jewelry or watchbands. Another kind of dermatitis can occur from frequent exposure to household detergents or other chemicals. Dermatitis causes itching, but scratching an affected area can make it worse. If you have dermatitis on your hands, wear cotton gloves under rubber gloves while you wash dishes or use household chemicals to prevent further irritation. Also, try to avoid using dyed or scented soaps and tissues, as they may aggravate your condition.

SYMPTOMS: *Patches of red, itchy skin*
• Tiny blisters on the affected area

	Rated on a scale of 1 to 10			Percentage of Pharmacists Who Most Often Recommend
	Most Effective	Speed Of Relief	Desirable Duration Of Relief	
Cortaid Maximum Strength	**8.6**	**8.1**	7.8	**50%**
Corticaine Maximum Strength	8.5	8.0	**7.9**	4%
Cortizone-10	**8.6**	8.0	7.8	33%
Kericort 10	8.3	7.8	7.6	•
Lanacort 10	8.3	7.9	7.7	2%
No Recommendation				11%

• Indicates that this product was recommended by less than 1% of pharmacists surveyed.
Bold type indicates the highest rating.

Pharmacists Say...

THESE PRODUCTS ARE USUALLY EFFECTIVE ONLY on minor skin irritations. When using these products, you should use a moisturizer regularly to increase the penetration of hydrocortisone and reduce itching.

GENERIC HYDROCORTISONE is as effective as and less expensive than name-brand versions.

HYDROCORTISONE should not be used on skin that is broken or bleeding.

THESE PRODUCTS MUST BE USED for three to four days before they'll achieve the best results.

See Your Doctor...

If the condition worsens, doesn't improve, or recurs after taking over-the-counter medication, contact your doctor.

See also *Dry Skin*

This section alphabetically lists all the products rated in the book. Under each product you will find its manufacturer, active Ingredients, dosage forms, and warnings, compiled as of September 1996.

A

A AND D MEDICATED DIAPER RASH OINTMENT WITH ZINC OXIDE
Schering-Plough HealthCare Products
Dosage Form: ointment
Active Ingredients: white petrolatum, zinc oxide
Warning: No other warnings other than those listed at the beginning of this section have been indicated by the manufacturer.

A-200 LICE KILLING SHAMPOO
Hogil Pharmaceutical Corporation
Dosage Form: shampoo
Active Ingredients: piperonyl butoxide, pyrethrum extract
Warning: Use with caution on persons allergic to ragweed. For external use only. Do not use near the eyes or permit contact with mucous membranes, such as the nose, mouth or vagina, as irritation may occur. Keep out of the eyes when rinsing hair. *Adults and children:* Close eyes tightly and do not open until product is rinsed out. Also protect children's eyes with wash cloth, towel or other suitable material or by a similar method. If product gets into the eyes, immediately flush with water. If skin irritation or infection is present or develops, discontinue use and consult a doctor. Consult a doctor if infestation of eyebrows or eyelashes occurs.

ABSORBINE FOOT CARE ANTIFUNGAL
W. F. Young, Inc.
Dosage Form: liquid spray, cream
Active Ingredient: tolnaftate
Warning: For external use only. Use only as directed. Avoid contact with the eyes and mucous membranes. If skin redness or irritation develops, if condition worsens, or does not improve within 7 days, or clears up and occurs again within a few days, discontinue use and consult a doctor. Do not use on children under 2 years of age except under the advice and supervision of a doctor. Do not apply to wounds, or to damaged, broken (open) or irritated skin. Do not bandage tightly. Do not use with a heating pad.

ABSORBINE JR. EXTRA STRENGTH LINIMENT
W. F. Young, Inc.
Dosage Form: liquid
Active Ingredient: menthol
Warning: Use only as directed. Replace cap firmly. If condition worsens, or symptoms persist for more than 7 days discontinue use and consult a doctor. Avoid contact with eyes. Do not use on children under 2 years of age

except under the advice and supervision of a doctor. Do not apply to wounds or damaged skin. Do not bandage.

ACTIFED COLD & ALLERGY
Warner Lambert Consumer Healthcare
Dosage Form: caplet, tablet
Active Ingredients: pseudoephedrine hydrochloride (HCl), triprolidine hydrochloride (HCl)
Warning: Do not exceed recommended dosage because at higher dosages, nervousness, dizziness, or sleeplessness may occur. If symptoms do not improve within 7 days or are accompanied by a fever, consult a doctor. Do not take this product if you have a breathing problem such as emphysema or chronic bronchitis, or if you have heart disease, high blood pressure, diabetes, thyroid disease, glaucoma or difficulty in urination due to enlargement of the prostate gland unless directed by a doctor. May cause excitability especially in children. May cause drowsiness; alcohol, sedatives, and tranquilizers may increase its drowsiness effect. Avoid alcoholic beverages while taking this product. Do not take this product if you are taking sedatives or tranquilizers without first consulting your doctor. Use caution while driving a motor vehicle or operating machinery. DRUG INTERACTION PRECAUTION: Do not use this product if you are now taking a prescription monoamine oxidase inhibitor (MAOI) (certain drugs for depression, psychiatric or emotional conditions, or Parkinson's disease) or for 2 weeks after stopping the MAOI drug. If you are uncertain if your prescription drug contains an MAOI, consult a health professional before taking this product.

ACTIFED COLD & SINUS
Warner Lambert Consumer Healthcare
Dosage Form: caplet, tablet
Active Ingredients: pseudoephedrine hydrochloride (HCl), triprolidine hydrochloride (HCl), acetaminophen
Warning: Do not exceed recommended dosage because at higher dosages, nervousness, dizziness, or sleeplessness may occur. Do not take this product for more than 10 days. If symptoms do not improve or are accompanied by a fever that lasts for more than 3 days or if new symptoms occur, consult a doctor. Do not take this product if you have a breathing problem such as emphysema or chronic bronchitis, or if you have heart disease, high blood pressure, diabetes, thyroid disease, glaucoma or difficulty in urination due to enlargement of the prostate gland unless directed by a doctor. May cause excitability especially in children. May cause drowsiness; alcohol, sedatives, and tranquilizers may increase its drowsiness effect. Avoid alcoholic beverages while taking this product. Do not take this product while taking sedatives or tranquilizers without first consulting your doctor. Use caution while driving a motor vehicle or operating machinery. Do not use with other products containing acetaminophen. DRUG INTERACTION PRECAUTION: Do

not use this product if you are now taking a prescription monoamine oxidase inhibitor (MAOI) (certain drugs for depression, psychiatric or emotional conditions, or Parkinson's disease) or for 2 weeks after stopping the MAOI drug. If you are uncertain if your prescription drug contains an MAOI, consult a health professional before taking this product.

ADVIL
Whitehall-Robins Healthcare
Dosage Form: caplet, tablet, gel caplet
Active Ingredient: ibuprofen
Warning: ASPIRIN SENSITIVE PATIENTS: Do not take this product if you have had a severe allergic reaction to aspirin, e.g.—asthma, swelling, shock or hives, because even though this product contains no aspirin or salicylates, cross-reactions may occur in patients allergic to aspirin. Do not take for pain for more than 10 days or for fever for more than 3 days unless directed by a doctor. If pain or fever persists or gets worse, if new symptoms occur, or if redness or swelling is present, consult a doctor. These could be signs of serious illness. If you are under a doctor's care for any serious condition, consult your doctor before taking this product. As with aspirin and acetaminophen, if you have any condition which requires you to take prescription drugs, or if you have had any problems or serious side effects from taking non-prescription pain relievers, do not take this product

For more information about the products' active ingredients, refer to the Glossary. Each active ingredient is listed there alphabetically with its function explained.

acetaminophen
Pain reliever

activated charcoal
Relieves symptoms of gas and diarrhea

allantoin
Helps stimulate tissue repair and soothe dry skin

aloe
Plant extract used to treat dry skin and sunburn

alpha-galactosidase (enzyme)
Relieves gas by promoting the breakdown of complex sugars in the small intestine

alum
Antibacterial and antifungal agent

aluminum hydroxide
Antacid

amethicone
Silicone oil used to treat dry skin

aspirin
Pain reliever and anti-inflammatory agent

attapulgite
Used to treat diarrhea

bacitracin
bacitracin zinc
Antibiotic used in ointments

benzalkonium chloride
Antiseptic agent

benzocaine
Anesthetic applied to the skin

benzoin tincture compound
Protective ingredient that keeps tissue from becoming irritated, so that it can heal

benzoyl peroxide
Antibacterial agent that promotes the shedding of upper skin layers; used in medications to treat acne

benzyl alcohol
Anesthetic

bisacodyl
Laxative

bismuth subsalicylate
Antidiarrheal agent that reduces fluid secretion in the gastrointestinal tract. By coating the stomach, this agent relieves symptoms of heartburn, indigestion, and upset stomach

boric acid
Antibacterial and antifungal agent

brompheniramine maleate
Antihistamine

butoconazole nitrate
Antifungal agent used to treat vaginal yeast infections

calamine
Relieves pain and itching of skin rashes and allergies

calcium carbonate
Antacid; also used in pain relievers to decrease stomach upset

calcium polycarbophil
Laxative

camphor
Antiseptic

capsaicin
Topical analgesic used in creams to relieve muscle and joint pain

carbamide peroxide
Antibacterial agent with emollient effects; used to soften earwax and to treat minor oral irritation

carboxymethylcellulose sodium
Used in eyedrops as a lubricant

casanthranol
Laxative

cascara sagrada
Laxative

cetalkonium chloride
Topical antibacterial agent

cetyl alcohol
Moisturizer used in lip glosses

chlorobutanol
Antimicrobial skin cleanser

chloroxylenol
Antibacterial agent

chlorpheniramine maleate
Antihistamine

cimetidine
Antiheartburn agent

clemastine fumarate
Antihistamine

clotrimazole
Antifungal agent

coal tar
coal tar solution
Used to treat skin and scalp conditions such as psoriasis and dandruff by reducing scale formation and increasing scale shedding

colloidal oatmeal
Used to soothe the skin

corn starch
Used in skin powders to prevent chafing, heat rash, and diaper rash

cyclizine hydrochloride (HCl)
Antihistamine used to treat nausea, vomiting, and motion sickness

dexbrompheniramine maleate
Antihistamine

dextran 70
Used to create artificial tears in eyedrops

dextromethorphan hydrobromide
Relieves coughs

dextromethorphan polistirex
Relieves coughs

dextrose
Decreases stomach and intestinal contractions to relieve symptoms of nausea and vomiting

dibasic sodium phosphate
Laxative

dimenhydrinate
Antihistamine used to relieve motion sickness

dimethicone
Silicone oil used to treat dry skin

diphenhydramine hydrochloride (HCl)
Antihistamine; also used in some sleeping pills

docusate calcium
Stool softener

docusate sodium
Stool softener

doxylamine succinate
Antihistamine. Also used in some sleeping pills.

dried aluminum
Antacid

dyclonine hydrochloride (HCl)
Anesthetic used to relieve sore throats

ethylhexyl p-methoxycinnamate
Protects skin from ultraviolet radiation

eugenol
Clove oil; used as an antiseptic for the skin and as a soothing ingredient in dental medications

famotidine
Antiheartburn agent

glycerin
Hydrating agent used in many medicines, including eyedrops, skin lotions, and hemorrhoid treatments

guaifenesin
Aids in the elimination of bronchial secretions that contribute to non-productive coughs

hydrocortisone
Mild steroid applied to the skin to relieve itching and swelling of many conditions

hydroxypropyl methylcellulose
Used to thicken eyedrops so they stay in your eyes

ibuprofen
Pain reliever and anti-inflammatory agent

isopropyl alcohol
Antiseptic and drying agent used externally

isopropyl myristate
Moisturizing agent used in lotions for dry skin and other topical products

ketoprofen
Pain reliever and anti-inflammatory agent

lanolin
Moisturizing agent

levulose
Decreases stomach and intestinal mobility to relieve symptoms of nausea and vomiting

lidocaine hydrochloride (HCl)
Anesthetic applied to the skin

loperamide hydrochloride (HCl)
Used to treat diarrhea

magaldrate
Antacid

magnesium carbonate
Antacid

magnesium hydroxide
Antacid

magnesium salicylate tetrahydrate
Pain reliever and anti-inflammatory agent

Ailments

This portion of the book contains an alphabetical listing and general description of common ailments and their symptoms, followed by the survey results for the relevant products, a "Pharmacists Say..." section, which contains useful information about the ailment and products, and a "See the Doctor..." section, which identifies warning signs that indicate when you need medical attention.

Five total attributes were chosen by the American Pharmaceutical Association and the Advisory Board pharmacists upon which to rate the products in this book. Of these, the three most relevant attributes were selected for rating the products within each ailment. This rating was based on a 1 to 10 scale, with 10 being the highest score.

The highest ratings have been highlighted in bold type. The 1 to 10 ratings for the attributes have been rounded to the nearest tenth of a point. The "Percentage Of Pharmacists Who Most Often Recommend" scores have been rounded to the nearest whole number. Because of this rounding, the sum total may not always equal exactly 100 percent.

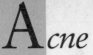

Acne

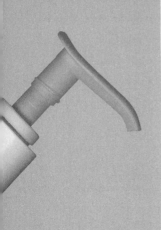

Acne is a skin disorder common to adolescents that's caused by inflammation of the sebaceous glands and hair follicles. If the sebaceous glands produce too much sebum (an oily substance that lubricates the skin), some of it can be trapped inside a follicle and become infected. Acne usually occurs on the face but may appear on the neck, back, chest, shoulders, and other areas. Acne ranges in severity from very mild forms, characterized by a few scattered blackheads and pimples, to severe acne, with large, painful pimples or cysts that lead to scarring. If you have acne, do not overscrub your skin; gentle washing twice a day with a mild soap should be enough. Acne-prone girls should avoid wearing foundation makeup and should always choose makeup products that are non-comedogenic, which means that they won't block your pores and cause more acne.

SYMPTOMS: *Whiteheads (raised pimples with a white plug at the top) • Blackheads (dark, closed pores; the darkness is caused by trapped melanin—a skin chemical that causes pigmentation—and not by dirt) • Red, swollen, cystlike lumps*

SOAPS AND FACIAL WASHES

	Rated on a scale of 1 to 10			Percentage Of Pharmacists Who Most Often Recommend
	Most Effective	**Speed Of Relief**	**Ease Of Use**	
Clean & Clear Deep Action Cream Cleanser	7.4	6.8	8.3	3%
Clearasil Antibacterial Soap	7.6	6.7	8.5	6%
Clearasil Daily Face Wash	7.8	7.0	8.7	7%
Fostex Acne Medication Cleansing Bar	7.8	6.8	8.6	3%
Neutrogena Oil-Free Acne Wash	8.0	7.0	8.6	9%
Oxy 10 Daily Face Wash	**8.6**	**7.3**	8.7	**45%**
Phisoderm Daily Skin Cleanser & Conditioner	7.6	6.8	**8.8**	16%
Propa pH Foaming Face Wash	7.5	6.8	8.3	•
Stri-Dex Antibacterial Cleansing Bar	7.9	7.0	8.3	1%
No Recommendation				11%

• *Indicates that this product was recommended by less than 1% of pharmacists surveyed.*
Bold type indicates the highest rating.

| | Rated on a scale of 1 to 10 | | | Percentage Of Pharmacists Who Most Often Recommend |
	Most Effective	Speed Of Relief	Desirable Duration Of Relief	
Clean & Clear Invisible Blemish Treatment	7.8	7.1	7.3	•
Clean & Clear Persa-Gel Extra Strength	8.4	7.5	7.5	10%
Clearasil Clearstick Maximum Strength	8.1	7.5	7.5	1%
Clearasil Ultra Pads with Aloe	7.9	7.4	7.3	2%
Clearasil Maximum Strength Vanishing or Tinted Cream	**8.9**	**7.9**	**8.0**	**33%**
Fostex 10% Benzoyl Peroxide Vanishing Gel	8.7	7.7	7.7	1%
Neutrogena Clear Pore Treatment	7.6	7.2	7.3	3%
Oxy 10 Maximum Strength Acne Treatment	8.8	**7.9**	7.8	32%
Stri-Dex Clear Gel	7.7	7.2	7.2	•
Stri-Dex Pads Maximum Strength	8.0	7.5	7.3	6%
No Recommendation				10%

• *Indicates that this product was recommended by less than 1% of pharmacists surveyed.*
Bold type indicates the highest rating.

Pharmacists Say...

ALTHOUGH USING A "MAXIMUM STRENGTH" PRODUCT may seem like the best idea, benzoyl peroxide is a very drying chemical and can irritate your skin, causing redness and peeling. Your best bet is to start with a "regular strength" (5% benzoyl peroxide) product and move up to a "maximum strength" (10%) product if your condition does not improve and you don't experience any skin irritation.

A GENERIC BENZOYL PEROXIDE SOAP OR WASH is just as effective as the more expensive name-brand products.

BENZOYL PEROXIDE products can bleach hair, bedding, and clothing, so be careful when you apply the medication, and make sure that it's completely dry before you change your clothes or go to bed.

DESPITE RUMORS TO THE CONTRARY, diet is probably not a significant factor in controlling acne.

See Your Doctor...

If you have mild acne that has not improved after four to eight weeks of using over-the-counter products, or if your acne is severe, contact your doctor.

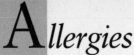

Allergies

Allergies are caused by excessive sensitivity to substances that your body believes are foreign. The immune system produces antibodies to attack these otherwise harmless substances, called "allergens." Common allergies include pollen, dust mites, mold, animal dander, foods, and medications. The allergic response can result in hay fever, hives, asthma, eczema, and, in some cases, life-threatening anaphylactic shock. The products in this section are rated on their ability to treat the symptoms described below.

SYMPTOMS: *Sneezing • Runny nose • Nasal or sinus congestion • Itchy eyes • Sinus headache • Cough*

For Adults

With sneezing, runny nose, itchy eyes:

ANTIHISTAMINES

	Rated on a scale of 1 to 10			Percentage Of Pharmacists Who Most Often Recommend
	Most Effective	Desirable Duration Of Relief	Minimal Side Effects	
Benadryl Allergy	**8.9**	7.3	5.7	24%
Chlor-Trimeton Allergy 12 Hour	8.7	**8.8**	7.1	29%
Dimetapp Allergy	8.5	7.7	7.0	6%
Tavist-1	8.7	8.4	**7.4**	**35%**
No Recommendation				7%

Bold type indicates the highest rating.

Pharmacists Say...

BECAUSE OVER-THE-COUNTER ANTIHISTAMINES cause drowsiness, you should first try a short-acting product (one that doesn't last for more than four hours) to assess how drowsy it makes you.

IF YOU HAVE PROBLEMS WITH DROWSINESS, try antihistamines containing chlorpheniramine such as Chlor-Trimeton. This ingredient is the least sedating of all the common over-the-counter antihistamines.

DO NOT CRUSH OR CHEW A LONG-ACTING PRODUCT. Swallow whole to prevent a sudden release of excessive medication.

SOME PEOPLE may become excitable or irritable when taking antihistamines. Children and the elderly are most likely to experience these side effects.

See also *Colds; Congestion: Head*

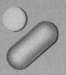

IF YOU HAVE GLAUCOMA, prostate disease, or breathing problems such as emphysema or chronic bronchitis, contact your pharmacist or doctor before taking any product containing an antihistamine.

ANTIHISTAMINES ARE AVAILABLE IN GENERIC BRANDS, which are just as effective and less expensive than name brands.

With sneezing, runny nose, itchy eyes:

DECONGESTANTS

	Rated on a scale of 1 to 10			Percentage Of Pharmacists Who Most Often Recommend
	Most Effective	**Desirable Duration Of Relief**	**Minimal Side Effects**	
Chlor-Trimeton Non-Drowsy Nasal Decongestant 4 Hour	8.2	7.1	7.7	•
Dimetapp Decongestant Non Drowsy Liqui-Gels	8.3	7.4	7.4	2%
Drixoral Non-Drowsy Nasal Decongestant 12 Hour Relief	8.5	8.3	7.5	5%
Efidac/24	8.4	**8.5**	7.3	11%
Sudafed Nasal Decongestant	**8.7**	7.6	**7.8**	**73%**
No Recommendation				9%

• Indicates that this product was recommended by less than 1% of pharmacists surveyed.
Bold type indicates the highest rating.

Pharmacists Say...

DECONGESTANTS ARE CONSIDERED NONSEDATING, because they don't contain antihistamines. Even though they may not be as effective as antihistamines in treating the sneezing, runny nose and itchy eyes due to allergies, they should be used when drowsiness could be a problem.

THE ACTIVE INGREDIENT IN THESE PRODUCTS is pseudoephedrine. This ingredient is available in generic products, which cost less and are just as effective as name brands.

PRODUCTS CONTAINING DECONGESTANTS may cause nervousness, dizziness, or sleeplessness.

IF YOU HAVE HEART DISEASE, high blood pressure, thyroid disease, diabetes, or prostate disease, contact your pharmacist or doctor before taking any product containing a decongestant.

DO NOT CRUSH OR CHEW A LONG-ACTING PRODUCT. Swallow whole to prevent a sudden release of excessive medication.

PEOPLE WHO ARE ELDERLY or who have never used decongestants should start with a short-acting product (one that doesn't last for more than four hours) to determine whether the medication causes excessive side effects.

continued on next page

*With sneezing, runny nose, itchy eyes, **and** head congestion:**

ANTIHISTAMINE, DECONGESTANT COMBINATIONS

	Rated on a scale of 1 to 10			Percentage Of Pharmacists Who Most Often Recommend
	Most Effective	**Desirable Duration Of Relief**	**Minimal Side Effects**	
Actifed Cold & Allergy	8.3	7.2	6.7	15%
Benadryl Allergy Decongestant	8.2	7.0	6.3	•
Chlor-Trimeton Allergy Decongestant 12 Hour	8.4	8.5	**7.4**	6%
Contac 12 Hour Cold	8.3	8.4	6.9	2%
Dimetapp 4-Hour Maximum Strength	8.4	7.9	7.3	16%
Drixoral Cold & Allergy 12 Hour Relief	8.5	**8.6**	7.3	8%
Sudafed Cold & Allergy	8.5	7.5	**7.4**	10%
Tavist-D	**8.8**	8.5	7.3	**41%**
No Recommendation				3%

* Head congestion can be either nasal or sinus congestion or both.

• Indicates that this product was recommended by less than 1% of pharmacists surveyed.
Bold type indicates the highest rating.

Pharmacists Say...

IF YOU HAVE A BREATHING PROBLEM such as emphysema or chronic bronchitis or have heart disease, high blood pressure, thyroid disease, diabetes, glaucoma, or prostate disease, contact your pharmacist or doctor before taking any product containing both an antihistamine and a decongestant.

SINCE THESE PRODUCTS contain both antihistamines and decongestants, you may experience the side effects of both medicines such as sedation, nervousness, or heart palpitations.

DO NOT CRUSH OR CHEW A LONG-ACTING PRODUCT. Swallow whole to prevent a sudden release of excessive medication.

GENERIC EQUIVALENTS are available for these products. They are less expensive and just as effective as the name brands.

With sneezing, runny nose, itchy eyes, head congestion, **and** *headache:*

ANTIHISTAMINE, DECONGESTANT, PAIN RELIEVER COMBINATIONS

	Rated on a scale of 1 to 10			Percentage Of Pharmacists Who Most Often Recommend
	Most Effective	**Desirable Duration Of Relief**	**Minimal Side Effects**	
Chlor-Trimeton Allergy•Sinus Headache	8.3	7.4	7.5	7%
Comtrex Maximum Strength Allergy-Sinus Treatment	8.3	7.5	7.3	10%
Coricidin 'D'	8.2	7.4	7.4	3%
Dristan Cold Multi-Symptom Formula	8.1	7.2	7.2	•
Sine-Off Sinus Medicine	8.2	7.4	7.3	1%
Sinutab Sinus Allergy Maximum Strength	8.4	7.6	7.6	10%
Triaminicin Cold, Allergy, Sinus Medicine	8.0	7.3	7.2	4%
Tylenol Allergy Sinus Maximum Strength	**8.6**	**7.7**	**7.8**	**45%**
No Recommendation				21%

* *Head congestion can be either nasal or sinus congestion or both.*

• *Indicates that this product was recommended by less than 1% of pharmacists surveyed.*

Bold type indicates the highest rating.

Pharmacists Say...

COMBINATION PRODUCTS CONTAIN MANY INGREDIENTS. If you take such a product you may be taking more medication than you need and subjecting yourself to unnecessary side effects. Treat only the symptoms that you actually have.

IF YOU HAVE A BREATHING PROBLEM such as emphysema or chronic bronchitis or have heart disease, high blood pressure, thyroid disease, diabetes, glaucoma, or prostate disease, contact your pharmacist or doctor before taking any product containing both an antihistamine and a decongestant.

GENERIC EQUIVALENTS are available for these products. They are less expensive and just as effective as the name brands.

continued on next page

For Children

With sneezing, runny nose, itchy eyes:

ANTIHISTAMINES

	Rated on a scale of 1 to 10			Percentage Of Pharmacists Who Most Often Recommend
	Most Effective	**Desirable Duration Of Relief**	**Speed Of Relief**	
Benadryl Allergy Liquid Medication	**8.9**	**7.8**	**8.2**	**62%**
Chlor-Trimeton Allergy	8.5	7.5	8.0	14%
Dimetapp Allergy Dye-Free Elixir	8.4	7.5	7.8	9%
Nolahist	7.4	7.3	7.5	•
No Recommendation				15%

• *Indicates that this product was recommended by less than 1% of pharmacists surveyed.*
Bold type indicates the highest rating.

Pharmacists Say...

IF YOUR CHILD HAS A HISTORY OF ASTHMA, chronic lung disease, or difficulty in urination, contact a doctor before giving your child any product containing an antihistamine.

ANTIHISTAMINES COMMONLY CAUSE DROWSINESS. However, in young children they may cause excitability.

SOME OF THESE PRODUCTS may contain alcohol or chemical dyes. Try to choose an alcohol-free and dye-free product for children.

GENERIC EQUIVALENTS are available for these products. They are less expensive and just as effective as the name brands.

With sneezing, runny nose, itchy eyes:

DECONGESTANTS

	Rated on a scale of 1 to 10			Percentage Of Pharmacists Who Most Often Recommend
	Most Effective	**Desirable Duration Of Relief**	**Ease Of Use**	
PediaCare Infants' Decongestant Drops	**8.7**	**7.8**	8.6	19%
Sudafed Children's Nasal Decongestant	**8.7**	**7.8**	**8.7**	**61%**
Triaminic AM Non-Drowsy Decongestant	8.4	7.6	8.4	10%
No Recommendation				9%

Bold type indicates the highest rating.

IF YOUR CHILD HAS A HISTORY OF HEART DISEASE, high blood pressure, diabetes, or thyroid disease, contact a doctor before giving your child any product containing a decongestant.

PRODUCTS CONTAINING DECONGESTANTS may cause nervousness, dizziness, or sleeplessness.

THE ACTIVE INGREDIENT IN THESE PRODUCTS is pseudo-ephedrine. This ingredient is available in generic products, which cost less and are just as effective as name brands.

DECONGESTANTS ARE CONSIDERED NONSEDATING, because they don't contain antihistamines. Even though they may not be as effective as antihistamines in treating the sneezing, runny nose and itchy eyes due to allergies, they should be used when drowsiness could be a problem.

If you don't obtain relief after several days of using these products, or if you can't tolerate the side effects of over-the-counter medications, contact your doctor.

Arthritis

Arthritis is a general term that refers to joint pain or stiffness. In simple terms, arthritis can be divided into two types: degenerative or osteoarthritis, and inflammatory arthritis. Osteoarthritis, the most common form, is caused by the breakdown of the normally smooth cartilage that lines the joints. Osteoarthritis usually involves the hips, knees, spine, hands, and feet, and causes stiffness or pain in the joints of affected areas. The inflammatory forms of arthritis are caused by infections, autoimmune diseases, or other medical problems and should be managed by a physician. For all arthritis sufferers, it's important not to let the muscles around the affected joints become weak from lack of use. If you're overweight, the strain on your joints can be relieved by weight loss. These over-the-counter products are only for the treatment of osteoarthritis.

SYMPTOMS: *Painful, swollen or stiff joints • Enlarged and "knobby" joints*

INTERNAL ANALGESICS

	Rated on a scale of 1 to 10			Percentage Of Pharmacists Who Most Often Recommend
	Most Effective	Speed Of Relief	Minimal Side Effects	
Advil	**8.7**	**8.1**	7.1	**54%**
Aleve	**8.7**	7.9	6.9	12%
Anacin Maximum Strength	7.9	7.8	6.9	1%
Ascriptin Maximum Strength	8.0	7.8	7.0	1%
Bayer Aspirin Extra Strength	8.2	7.8	6.7	1%
Bufferin Arthritis Strength	8.0	7.8	7.0	3%
Ecotrin Maximum Strength	8.0	7.1	7.1	4%
Motrin IB	**8.7**	**8.1**	7.1	10%
Nuprin Pain Relief Formula	**8.7**	**8.1**	7.2	•
Orudis KT	8.5	7.8	6.8	5%
Tylenol Extra Strength	6.7	7.1	**8.5**	4%
No Recommendation				6%

• *Indicates that this product was recommended by less than 1% of pharmacists surveyed.*
Bold type indicates the highest rating.

See also *Bursitis/Tendinitis*

TYLENOL OR GENERIC ACETAMINOPHEN is the safest over-the-counter product for pain relief and is recommended for the treatment of osteoarthritis by the American College of Rheumatology. However, if your pain is not relieved or there is significant inflammation, try an anti-inflammatory medication such as aspirin, ibuprofen, naproxen, etc., but be sure to take these medications with food, to avoid upsetting your stomach.

IF YOU ARE TAKING OTHER MEDICATION, check with your pharmacist or doctor about possible interactions before you take any of these products.

ADVIL, NUPRIN, AND MOTRIN IB are identical products containing 200 mg of ibuprofen.

IF YOU HAVE A HISTORY OF PEPTIC ULCERS, bleeding disorders, kidney disease, or asthma, contact your doctor before taking an over-the-counter anti-inflammatory medication such as aspirin, ibuprofen, naproxen, etc.

GENERIC EQUIVALENTS are available for these products. They are less expensive and just as effective as the name brands.

continued on next page

| | Rated on a scale of 1 to 10 | | | Percentage Of Pharmacists Who Most Often Recommend |
	Most Effective	Speed Of Relief	Minimal Side Effects	
Absorbine Jr. Extra Strength Liniment	6.6	7.0	7.8	•
ArthriCare Triple Medicated Pain Relieving Rub	7.2	7.3	7.6	2%
Arthritis Hot Pain Relief Creme	7.0	7.3	7.4	•
Aspercreme	6.8	7.1	8.2	10%
BenGay Arthritis Formula	7.2	7.5	7.8	9%
Capzasin-P	8.5	7.1	7.3	**27%**
Heet Pain Relieving Liniment	7.4	**7.6**	7.3	1%
Icy Hot	7.1	7.5	7.8	4%
Myoflex External Analgesic Creme	7.2	7.2	**8.3**	15%
Zostrix-HP High Potency	**8.6**	7.2	7.3	20%
No Recommendation				13%

• Indicates that this product was recommended by less than 1% of pharmacists surveyed.

Bold type indicates the highest rating.

Pharmacists Say...

THESE MEDICATIONS MAY CAUSE IRRITATION OR BURNING and should not be used on broken or inflamed skin. Be sure to wash your hands thoroughly after using these products, and strictly avoid contact with the eyes or other mucous membranes such as your mouth, nostrils, and genitals. If excessive skin irritation occurs, stop using the product immediately.

IF YOU'RE USING an external pain-relieving rub or cream, don't use a heating pad on the same area! Severe burns may occur.

PRODUCTS CONTAINING CAPSAICIN, such as Capzasin-P and Zostrix-HP, provide the greatest relief but may take several weeks to produce results. Initially patients may experience an uncomfortable burning sensation, which subsides with continued use. These products also tend to be more expensive than other rubs.

At the onset of joint pain or discomfort, contact your doctor to determine the exact cause of the symptoms. Minor pain associated with osteoarthritis that is not relieved after two weeks of taking the maximum recommended dose of over-the-counter medications should be evaluated by your doctor. Fever, redness, or tenderness at the site of the joint pain warrants immediate attention, as it may indicate a more serious condition. Furthermore, patients who develop abdominal pain or nausea or who have difficulty breathing should discontinue use of the product and contact their doctor immediately.

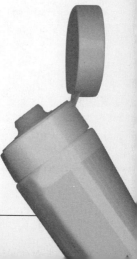

Athlete's Foot

Athlete's foot is a harmless but irritating condition caused by a fungus that thrives in warm, moist areas. Athlete's foot is slightly contagious. In addition to the antifungal medications listed here, you should be sure to dry between your toes carefully after swimming or bathing; wear cotton socks and change them daily, or wear open sandals or shoes; and air out your shoes well when you're not wearing them.

SYMPTOMS: *Red, flaky, itchy skin between and under toes, especially the fourth and fifth toes • Unpleasant smell • Skin is white and soggy when moist*

	Rated on a scale of 1 to 10			Percentage Of Pharmacists Who Most Often Recommend
	Most Effective	Speed Of Relief	Ease Of Use	
Absorbine Foot Care Antifungal	7.0	6.8	8.4	•
Cruex Antifungal Cream	7.3	6.8	8.2	•
Desenex Antifungal Ointment	7.3	6.9	8.1	1%
Desenex Prescription Strength Liquid Spray	7.7	7.2	8.2	2%
Dr. Scholl's Athlete's Foot	7.4	7.0	8.1	•
Lotrimin Antifungal AF Cream	**9.2**	**8.0**	**8.6**	**70%**
Micatin	8.7	7.8	8.5	15%
Mycelex OTC Antifungal Cream	8.8	7.8	8.5	2%
Tinactin Antifungal Cream	8.3	7.5	8.5	9%
Zeasorb-AF	7.6	6.9	8.3	•
No Recommendation				1%

• Indicates that this product was recommended by less than 1% of pharmacists surveyed.
Bold type indicates the highest rating.

BE PATIENT EXPECTING RESULTS. You should use the product as directed, for 1 to 2 weeks after the symptoms are gone. Athlete's foot can be cured if you are thorough and persist long enough.

THE ANTIFUNGAL CREAMS are probably the best form to use for initial treatment, while sprays and powders are best for prevention and maintenance.

THE ACTIVE INGREDIENTS in most medications—clotrimazole or miconazole—are usually equally effective in treating athlete's foot. These ingredients are also used in treatments for vaginal yeast infection. If you're interested in saving money, you can purchase generic vaginal creams used as treatment for yeast infections and use them without the applicator. (For example, a generic equivalent of Gyne-Lotrimin or Monistat 7 usually provides a 45 g tube for the price of a 12 g tube of Lotrimin AF.)

Patients with diabetes or other vascular problems should consult their doctor if they experience any type of foot problem. If you have athlete's foot that doesn't respond to over-the-counter medications, or if irritation occurs as a result of these products, contact your doctor.

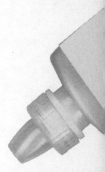

Backache

Most backaches occur as a result of musculoskeletal injury or stress. Recurrent back pain may be a symptom of disc disease or arthritis. The best thing to do for backaches is prevent them: be sure that you lift heavy objects correctly (keep your back straight and bend your knees); wear low-heeled shoes; sleep on a firm mattress; and maintain correct posture when sitting and standing. Self-help treatments for backache include applying ice to the painful area within the first 24 hours after injury and then heat afterward; lying flat on your back; and gentle massage.

S Y M P T O M S : *Back pain and stiffness*

INTERNAL PAIN RELIEVERS

	Rated on a scale of 1 to 10			Percentage Of Pharmacists Who Most Often Recommend
	Most Effective	**Speed Of Relief**	**Minimal Side Effects**	
Advil	**8.7**	8.1	7.1	**45%**
Aleve	**8.7**	8.0	6.9	18%
Ascriptin Maximum Strength	7.9	7.8	7.0	•
Backache Maximum Strength Relief	8.1	7.9	7.0	•
Bayer Aspirin Extra Strength	7.9	7.8	6.8	•
Bufferin Extra Strength	7.9	7.8	7.0	1%
Doan's Extra Strength	7.5	7.6	7.0	2%
Ecotrin Maximum Strength	7.7	7.1	7.3	•
Motrin IB	**8.7**	**8.2**	7.1	11%
Nuprin Pain Relief Formula	**8.7**	**8.2**	7.1	1%
Orudis KT	8.6	8.0	6.8	4%
Tylenol Extra Strength	7.0	7.2	**8.6**	3%
No Recommendation				15%

• *Indicates that this product was recommended by less than 1% of pharmacists surveyed.*
Bold type indicates the highest rating.

TYLENOL OR GENERIC ACETAMINOPHEN is the safest over-the-counter product for pain relief. However, if your pain is not relieved or there is significant inflammation, try an anti-inflammatory medication such as aspirin, ibuprofen, naproxen, etc., but be sure to take these medications with food, to avoid upsetting your stomach.

IF YOU ARE TAKING OTHER MEDICATION, check with your pharmacist or doctor about possible interactions before you take any of these products.

ADVIL, NUPRIN, AND MOTRIN IB are identical products containing 200 mg of ibuprofen.

IF YOU HAVE A HISTORY OF PEPTIC ULCERS, bleeding disorders, kidney disease, or asthma, contact your doctor before taking an over-the-counter anti-inflammatory medication such as aspirin, ibuprofen, naproxen, etc.

GENERIC EQUIVALENTS are available for these products. They are less expensive and just as effective as the name brands.

EXTERNAL PAIN RELIEVERS

| | Rated on a scale of 1 to 10 | | | Percentage Of Pharmacists Who Most Often Recommend |
	Most Effective	Speed Of Relief	Minimal Side Effects	
Absorbine Jr. Extra Strength Liniment	7.1	7.4	7.9	1%
Aspercreme	7.2	7.3	**8.1**	13%
BenGay Original Formula	7.6	7.8	7.9	7%
Capzasin-P	**7.9**	7.1	7.3	16%
Flex-All 454 Maximum Strength	7.8	**7.9**	**8.1**	**21%**
Heet Pain Relieving Liniment	7.5	7.7	7.5	1%
Icy Hot	7.5	**7.9**	7.8	8%
Thera-Gesic Extra Strength	7.7	**7.9**	8.0	6%
Therapeutic Mineral Ice	7.5	7.8	8.0	11%
No Recommendation				23%

Bold type indicates the highest rating.

continued on next page

THESE MEDICATIONS MAY CAUSE IRRITATION OR BURNING and should not be used on broken or inflamed skin. Be sure to wash your hands thoroughly after using these products, and strictly avoid contact with the eyes or other mucous membranes such as your mouth, nostrils, and genitals. If excessive skin irritation occurs, stop using the product immediately.

IF YOU'RE USING AN EXTERNAL PAIN-RELIEVING RUB or cream, don't use a heating pad on the same area! Severe burns can occur.

PRODUCTS CONTAINING CAPSAICIN, such as Capzasin-P, provide the greatest relief but may take several weeks to produce results. Initially, patients may experience an uncomfortable burning sensation, which subsides with continued use. These products also tend to be more expensive than other rubs.

There are many causes of back pain, some of which are quite serious. If you experience sharp pain that radiates into your buttocks or legs, if you have weakness or numbness in your legs, or if you are unable to control your bladder or bowels, contact your doctor immediately. Fever, chills, painful urination, or blood in the urine that are associated with back pain may indicate an underlying infection and warrant immediate attention. If your backache doesn't improve after one or two weeks of rest, warm baths, and use of over-the-counter products, or if your backache occurs frequently, contact your doctor. Elderly patients with a sudden onset of back pain should contact their doctor immediately. Furthermore, patients who develop abdominal pain or nausea or who have difficulty breathing should discontinue use of the product and contact their doctor immediately.

Bee Sting

After a bee sting, check to see if a stinger remains. If present, remove it without using tweezers if possible, which can squeeze more venom into the skin. Instead, gently press the area with the index fingers of both hands to push the stinger out. Wash the bite with soap and water, then use ice packs or cold compresses to decrease the swelling and pain.

SYMPTOMS: *Pain or swelling at location of bite • Redness, itching, and burning • Multiple stings may cause headache, muscle cramps, or fever*

	Rated on a scale of 1 to 10			Percentage Of Pharmacists Who Most Often Recommend
	Most Effective	**Speed Of Relief**	**Ease Of Use**	
Americaine Topical Anesthetic Spray	7.8	8.2	**9.0**	9%
Bactine First Aid	7.0	7.5	8.5	7%
Cortaid Maximum Strength	7.5	7.0	8.5	13%
Cortizone-10	7.4	7.0	8.5	11%
Lanacort 10	7.5	6.9	8.6	1%
Solarcaine Medicated First Aid	7.7	8.1	8.8	9%
Sting-Eze	8.2	8.1	8.7	9%
Sting-Kill	**8.3**	**8.5**	8.5	**23%**
No Recommendation				15%

Bold type indicates the highest rating.

Pharmacists Say...

TRY TO TAKE AN ORAL ANTIHISTAMINE such as Benadryl or an equivalent generic as soon as possible after a sting, to help reduce the swelling. See 'General Warnings' (page xiii) regarding antihistamines.

IF YOU HAVE ANY PAIN associated with the sting, take Tylenol or a generic acetaminophen product.

continued on next page

IF OVER-THE-COUNTER PRODUCTS are not available, applying a paste of baking soda and water to the sting can provide relief.

GENERIC EQUIVALENTS are available for these products. They are less expensive and just as effective as the name brands.

See Your Doctor...

If you have a history of allergic reactions to bee stings or if you are stung and experience lightheadedness, dizziness, nausea, vomiting, lethargy, shortness of breath, or flushed or clammy skin, contact your doctor immediately. Bee stings that result in extensive swelling or redness should also be seen by a doctor.

Boils

Boils occur when a hair follicle becomes infected with bacteria, which causes pain and swelling. Boils will usually drain of their own accord. You can relieve pain and hasten drainage by applying a hot, moist compress to the area every few hours.

SYMPTOMS: *A red, tender lump that swells and fills with pus*

| | Rated on a scale of 1 to 10 | | | Percentage Of Pharmacists Who Most Often Recommend |
	Most Effective	Speed Of Relief	Minimal Side Effects	
Baciguent	6.6	6.1	8.6	1%
Boil Ease	**7.4**	**7.0**	8.6	**52%**
Neosporin Original	6.9	6.2	**8.7**	24%
No Recommendation				23%

Bold type indicates the highest rating.

Pharmacists Say...

AFTER A BOIL DRAINS, continue to apply warm compresses and apply an antibiotic ointment to prevent infection.

BECAUSE OF ITS ACTIVE INGREDIENT, benzocaine, Boil Ease will be more effective relieving the pain associated with boils, while Baciguent and Neosporin, both antibiotics, will be more effective preventing infection after the boil drains.

See Your Doctor...

If you have multiple boils that recur frequently or if you have boils associated with fever, chills, or excessive pain, redness, or streaking in the affected area, contact your doctor.

Burns

Burns are a common injury and are classified by the degree of damage to the skin. First-degree burns involve the outermost layers of skin and are red and painful. These types of burns are usually caused by short exposure to a hot substance, such as picking up a hot pan or brief exposure to steam. Second-degree burns are a deeper burn that leads to the formation of blisters. Third-degree burns are deeper still, damaging all the layers of the skin, including the nerve endings. Third-degree burns are painless, and appear white or charred. First-degree burns are best treated by applying cold compresses of water, milk, or oatmeal to the affected area until the pain is gone. These over-the-counter products are only for the treatment of first-degree burns involving a small area of skin.

SYMPTOMS OF MINOR BURNS:
Redness • Pain

TO RELIEVE PAIN

	Rated on a scale of 1 to 10			Percentage Of Pharmacists Who Most Often Recommend
	Most Effective	**Speed Of Relief**	**Ease Of Use**	
Bactine First Aid	7.3	7.6	8.6	3%
Dermoplast Pain Relieving Spray	**8.6**	**8.6**	**9.0**	**33%**
Foille Medicated First Aid	8.1	8.2	8.7	16%
Lanacane Maximum Strength Spray Medication	8.1	8.3	8.7	9%
Solarcaine Medicated First Aid	8.4	8.5	**9.0**	31%
No Recommendation				8%

Bold type indicates the highest rating.

	Rated on a scale of 1 to 10			Percentage Of Pharmacists Who Most Often Recommend
	Most Effective	Speed Of Relief	Ease Of Use	
Cortaid Maximum Strength	**8.4**	8.0	**8.4**	**42%**
Cortizone-10	**8.4**	**8.1**	**8.4**	30%
No Recommendation				28%

Bold type indicates the highest rating.

Pharmacists Say...

IF THE BURN IS PAINFUL, you may want to try a spray first, as applying a cream or lotion may make the burn hurt more. You can also take ibuprofen or acetaminophen for the pain. See 'General Warnings' (page xiii) regarding anti-inflammatory medications.

IT'S VERY IMPORTANT to keep burns clean and free from infection as they heal. Be sure to wash the area well, gently pat it dry, and apply an antibiotic ointment, such as bacitracin.

See Your Doctor...

The only burns that you should treat at home are small first-degree burns. All extensive burns and any burn with blistering should be seen by a doctor.

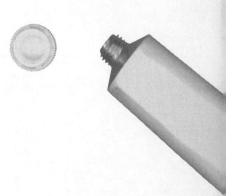

Bursitis/Tendinitis

Bursitis is caused by inflammation of the bursa, a soft sac of lubricating fluid (usually near a joint) that acts as a cushion between skin and bones or tendons and bones. If the bursa is irritated, it becomes swollen and painful. Bursitis commonly occurs in the shoulder, elbow, hip, and knee. If you have bursitis, you should keep all pressure off the swollen area and avoid repetitive activity at that joint.

Tendinitis occurs when a tendon (the tissue that connects muscles to bones) becomes inflamed or torn. Tendons are slow to heal, so the pain may persist for several weeks. Tennis elbow and golfer's elbow are common forms of tendinitis caused by overexertion in sports; however, tendinitis can develop in other joints such as the knee, wrist, or shoulder. If you have tendinitis, prolonged rest may be necessary to allow the inflamed tendon to heal.

S Y M P T O M S : *Pain and swelling around a joint*

	Rated on a scale of 1 to 10			Percentage Of Pharmacists Who Most Often Recommend
	Most Effective	**Speed Of Relief**	**Minimal Side Effects**	
Advil	**8.7**	**8.2**	7.1	**50%**
Aleve	**8.7**	8.0	6.9	12%
Anacin Maximum Strength	7.9	7.9	6.8	1%
Ascriptin Maximum Strength	7.9	7.8	6.9	•
Bayer Aspirin Extra Strength	8.0	7.9	6.7	2%
Bufferin Arthritis Strength	7.9	7.8	6.8	1%
Ecotrin Maximum Strength	7.8	7.2	7.0	•
Motrin IB	**8.7**	**8.2**	7.2	14%
Nuprin Pain Relief Formula	**8.7**	**8.2**	7.1	•
Orudis KT	8.6	8.0	6.9	8%
Tylenol Extra Strength	6.3	6.9	**8.7**	1%
No Recommendation				10%

• Indicates that this product was recommended by less than 1% of pharmacists surveyed.
Bold type indicates the highest rating.

See also *Arthritis*

TYLENOL OR GENERIC ACETAMINOPHEN is the safest over-the-counter product for pain relief. However, if your pain is not relieved or there is significant inflammation, try an anti-inflammatory medication such as aspirin, ibuprofen, naproxen, etc., but be sure to take these medications with food, to avoid upsetting your stomach.

IF YOU ARE TAKING OTHER MEDICATION, check with your pharmacist or doctor about possible interactions before you take any of these products.

ADVIL, NUPRIN, AND MOTRIN IB are identical products containing 200 mg of ibuprofen.

IF YOU HAVE A HISTORY OF PEPTIC ULCERS, bleeding disorders, kidney disease, or asthma, contact your doctor before taking an over-the-counter anti-inflammatory medication such as aspirin, ibuprofen, naproxen, etc.

PATIENTS MAY OBTAIN additional relief by applying ice two to three times daily.

GENERIC EQUIVALENTS are available for these products. They are less expensive and just as effective as the name brands.

At the onset of joint pain or discomfort, contact your doctor to determine the exact cause of the symptoms. Minor pain that is not relieved after two weeks of taking the maximum recommended dose of over-the-counter medications should be evaluated by your doctor. Fever, redness, and tenderness at the sight of the joint pain warrants immediate attention, as it may indicate a more serious condition. Furthermore, patients who develop abdominal pain or nausea or who have difficulty breathing should discontinue use of the product and contact their doctor immediately.

Canker Sores

Canker sores are a common condition in which small painful ulcers develop in the mouth. The cause of canker sores remains unknown; however, they are associated with certain diseases, stress, and vitamin deficiencies. Additionally, some women may develop canker sores before their menstrual cycle. Canker sores are not contagious and usually go away within one to two weeks. If you have canker sores, avoid hot, spicy, or acidic foods and beverages.

SYMPTOMS: *Painful white or pale yellow spots with red borders*

	Rated on a scale of 1 to 10			Percentage Of Pharmacists Who Most Often Recommend
	Most Effective	**Desirable Duration Of Relief**	**Speed Of Relief**	
Anbesol Maximum Strength	8.5	7.6	6.9	9%
Gly-Oxide	7.3	7.5	6.6	14%
Kank-A Professional Strength Mouth Sore Medication	8.1	7.7	6.9	5%
Orabase Gel Oral Analgesic Protective Gel	7.3	7.1	6.8	4%
Orabase-B With Benzocaine	**8.6**	**8.2**	**7.6**	**30%**
Orajel Mouth-Aid	8.5	7.9	7.3	3%
SensoGARD Canker Sore Relief	7.4	7.1	6.8	2%
Tanac No Sting	7.9	7.5	6.7	4%
Zilactin Medicated Gel	8.0	7.8	7.4	25%
No Recommendation				5%

Bold type indicates the highest rating.

Pharmacists Say...

YOU CAN HELP CANKER SORES to heal by rinsing your mouth with a solution of equal parts of hydrogen peroxide and water.

YOU'LL GET THE BEST RESULTS if you carefully dry the area before applying the product, and avoid eating or drinking directly after application.

See also *Cold Sores*

IN ADDITION TO THE MEASURES DESCRIBED HERE, acetaminophen or ibuprofen can be used to help alleviate pain.
See 'General Warnings' (page xiii) regarding anti-inflammatory
medications.

See Your Doctor...

*If the sores persist for more than seven to ten days and
there is no relief provided by medications listed in this
section, consult your doctor.*

Chapped Lips

Chapped lips occur when sufficient moisture isn't available to the outer tissues of the lips. This can be caused by dehydration or by overexposure to the elements, such as cold dry air, sun, or wind. The best protection against chapped lips is to use lip balm and drink plenty of fluids.

SYMPTOMS: *Dry, cracked lips*

| | Rated on a scale of 1 to 10 | | | Percentage Of Pharmacists Who Most Often Recommend |
	Most Effective	Ease Of Use	Speed Of Relief	
Blistex Lip Medex	8.5	8.6	8.4	9%
Blistex Medicated Lip Ointment	8.2	8.8	8.3	15%
Carmex Lip Balm	**8.7**	8.7	**8.6**	**42%**
ChapStick Lip Balm	7.6	8.9	8.0	14%
Orabase Lip	8.2	8.8	8.2	0%
Vaseline Lip Therapy	8.2	**9.0**	8.2	12%
No Recommendation				8%

WITH SUNSCREEN

| | Rated on a scale of 1 to 10 | | | Percentage Of Pharmacists Who Most Often Recommend |
	Most Effective	Ease Of Use	Speed Of Relief	
Blistex Medicated Lip Balm	8.4	8.3	9.0	22%
ChapStick Sunblock 15	**8.7**	**8.5**	9.0	**50%**
Vaseline Lip Therapy Advanced Formula	8.6	8.4	**9.1**	17%
No Recommendation				11%

Bold type indicates the highest rating.

Pharmacists Say...

THESE PRODUCTS SHOULD BE APPLIED frequently to help heal and prevent chapped lips.

IT'S IMPORTANT TO REMEMBER that lips are as susceptible to sunburn as other areas of the body. To prevent sun-damaged lips, be sure to use a lip balm with sunscreen throughout the year.

See Your Doctor...

Chapped lips do not require medical attention.

Colds

What we call "the common cold" is actually a group of minor illnesses caused by one of nearly 200 different viruses. The symptoms of a cold depend on which virus you have but may include any or all of the symptoms listed below. If you have body pains and a high fever, you may have the flu or other infection instead of a cold. Despite common belief, you can't avoid colds by taking super-doses of vitamins, and colds are not caused by wet feet or exposure to drafts. Your best bet is to wash your hands frequently and avoid hand-to-mouth contact if you've been around someone who is infected. If you have a cold, you should stay home to rest and to ensure that you don't infect others. Using a vaporizer or humidifier to increase moisture in the air may provide additional relief. Be sure to drink plenty of fluids to maintain the balance of liquid in your body.

SYMPTOMS: *Sneezing • Runny nose • Nasal or chest congestion • Coughing • Slight fever*

For Adults

With sneezing, runny nose, watery eyes:

ANTIHISTAMINES

	Rated on a scale of 1 to 10			Percentage Of Pharmacists Who Most Often Recommend
	Most Effective	**Speed Of Relief**	**Desirable Duration Of Relief**	
Benadryl Allergy	**8.6**	8.1	6.9	24%
Chlor-Trimeton Allergy 12 Hour	8.4	7.9	**8.6**	25%
Dimetapp Allergy	8.2	7.8	7.6	9%
Tavist-1	**8.6**	**8.2**	**8.6**	**36%**
No Recommendation				6%

Bold type indicates the highest rating.

Pharmacists Say...

ANTIHISTAMINES may not be as effective in treating the common cold as they are in treating allergies.

BECAUSE OVER-THE-COUNTER ANTIHISTAMINES cause drowsiness, you should first try a short-acting product (one that doesn't last for more than four hours) to assess how drowsy it makes you.

continued on next page

See also *Congestion: Chest; Congestion: Head; Coughs; Fever; Sore Throat*

IF YOU HAVE PROBLEMS with drowsiness, try antihistamines containing chlorpheniramine such as Chlor-Trimeton. This ingredient is the least sedating of all the common over-the-counter antihistamines.

ANTIHISTAMINES ARE AVAILABLE IN GENERIC BRANDS, which are just as effective and less expensive than name brands.

IF YOU HAVE GLAUCOMA, prostate disease, or breathing problems such as emphysema or chronic bronchitis, contact your pharmacist or doctor before taking any product containing an antihistamine.

DO NOT CRUSH OR CHEW A LONG-ACTING PRODUCT. Swallow whole to prevent a sudden release of excessive medication.

SOME PEOPLE may become excitable or irritable when taking antihistamines. Children and the elderly are most likely to experience these side effects.

*With sneezing, runny nose, watery eyes, and head congestion:**

ANTIHISTAMINE, DECONGESTANT COMBINATIONS

	Rated on a scale of 1 to 10			Percentage Of Pharmacists Who Most Often Recommend
	Most Effective	Speed Of Relief	Desirable Duration Of Relief	
Actifed Cold & Allergy	8.3	7.9	7.2	12%
Benadryl Allergy Decongestant	8.2	7.8	7.0	1%
Chlor-Trimeton Allergy Decongestant 12 Hour	8.4	7.7	**8.5**	5%
Contac 12 Hour Cold	8.2	7.6	8.3	3%
Dimetapp 4-Hour Maximum Strength	8.4	8.0	7.8	15%
Drixoral Cold & Allergy 12 Hour Relief	8.4	7.8	8.3	10%
Sudafed Cold & Allergy	8.4	**8.1**	7.3	11%
Tavist-D	**8.7**	8.0	8.4	**38%**
No Recommendation				4%

*Head congestion can be either nasal or sinus congestion or both.
Bold type indicates the highest rating.

Pharmacists Say...

IF YOU HAVE A BREATHING PROBLEM such as emphysema or chronic bronchitis or have heart disease, high blood pressure, thyroid disease, diabetes, glaucoma, or prostate disease, contact your pharmacist or doctor before taking any product containing both an antihistamine and a decongestant.

SINCE THESE PRODUCTS contain both antihistamines and decongestants, you may experience the side effects of both medicines such as sedation, nervousness, or heart palpitations.

DO NOT CRUSH OR CHEW A LONG-ACTING PRODUCT. Swallow whole to prevent a sudden release of excessive medication.

GENERIC EQUIVALENTS are available for these products. They are less expensive and just as effective as the name brands.

With sneezing, runny nose, watery eyes, head congestion, **and** headache:*

ANTIHISTAMINE, DECONGESTANT, PAIN RELIEVER COMBINATIONS

	Rated on a scale of 1 to 10			Percentage Of Pharmacists Who Most Often Recommend
	Most Effective	Speed Of Relief	Desirable Duration Of Relief	
Actifed Cold & Sinus	8.0	7.7	7.5	4%
Alka-Seltzer Plus Cold Medicine Liqui-Gels	8.0	**8.3**	7.3	12%
Benadryl Allergy/Cold	7.9	7.6	7.0	1%
Coricidin 'D'	7.9	7.6	7.4	3%
Dimetapp Allergy Sinus	8.1	7.6	7.8	11%
Dristan Cold Multi-Symptom Formula	7.8	7.7	7.3	2%
Drixoral Cold & Flu 12 Hour Relief	**8.3**	7.7	**8.1**	**20%**
Sinarest Extra Strength	7.6	7.5	7.0	1%
TheraFlu Flu and Cold Medicine Original Formula	8.2	**8.3**	7.4	18%
Tylenol Allergy Sinus NightTime Maximum Strength	8.2	7.7	7.3	8%
No Recommendation				20%

*Head congestion can be either nasal or sinus congestion or both.
Bold type indicates the highest rating.

Pharmacists Say...

COMBINATION PRODUCTS CONTAIN MANY INGREDIENTS. If you take such a product you may be taking more medication than you need and subjecting yourself to unnecessary side effects. Treat only the symptoms that you actually have.

continued on next page

IF YOU HAVE A BREATHING PROBLEM such as emphysema or chronic bronchitis or have heart disease, high blood pressure, thyroid disease, diabetes, glaucoma, or prostate disease, contact your pharmacist or doctor before taking any product containing both an antihistamine and a decongestant.

DO NOT CRUSH OR CHEW A LONG-ACTING PRODUCT. Swallow whole to prevent a sudden release of excessive medication.

GENERIC EQUIVALENTS are available for these products. They are less expensive and just as effective as the name brands.

With head congestion* only:

DECONGESTANTS

	Rated on a scale of 1 to 10			Percentage Of Pharmacists Who Most Often Recommend
	Most Effective	**Speed Of Relief**	**Desirable Duration Of Relief**	
Chlor-Trimeton Non-Drowsy Nasal Decongestant 4 Hour	8.3	8.1	6.9	•
Dimetapp Decongestant Non Drowsy Liqui-Gels	8.3	7.9	7.3	1%
Drixoral Non-Drowsy Nasal Decongestant 12-Hour Relief	8.6	7.7	**8.3**	7%
Efidac/24	8.4	7.7	**8.3**	8%
Sudafed Nasal Decongestant	**8.8**	**8.4**	7.2	**80%**
No Recommendation				5%

*Head congestion can be either nasal or sinus congestion or both.
• Indicates that this product was recommended by less than 1% of pharmacists surveyed.
Bold type indicates the highest rating.

Pharmacists Say...

THE ACTIVE INGREDIENT IN THESE PRODUCTS is pseudo-ephedrine. It is available in generic products, which cost less and are just as effective as name brands.

PRODUCTS CONTAINING DECONGESTANTS may cause nervousness, dizziness, or sleeplessness.

IF YOU HAVE HEART DISEASE, high blood pressure, thyroid disease, diabetes, or prostate disease, contact your pharmacist or doctor before taking any product containing a decongestant.

PEOPLE WHO ARE ELDERLY or who have never used decongestants should start with a short-acting product (one that doesn't last for more than four hours) to determine whether the medication causes excessive side effects.

IF YOU CAN'T TOLERATE THE SIDE EFFECTS of decongestants, try using saline or decongestant nasal sprays as an alternative treatment. These sprays are less likely to cause side effects such as anxiety, increased blood pressure, and heart palpitations. However, be aware that using decongestant nasal sprays for more than three days can make your nasal congestion worse.

DO NOT CRUSH OR CHEW A LONG-ACTING PRODUCT. Swallow whole to prevent a sudden release of excessive medication.

With head congestion **and** *headache:*

DECONGESTANT, PAIN RELIEVER COMBINATIONS

	Rated on a scale of 1 to 10			Percentage Of Pharmacists Who Most Often Recommend
	Most Effective	**Speed Of Relief**	**Desirable Duration Of Relief**	
Advil Cold & Sinus	**8.7**	**8.2**	7.7	**38%**
Dristan Sinus	8.2	7.9	7.5	•
Motrin IB Sinus	**8.7**	8.1	7.7	4%
Sinarest No Drowsiness	7.9	7.8	7.4	0%
Sine-Aid Maximum Strength	8.1	7.8	7.6	3%
Sinutab Sinus No Drowsiness Maximum Strength	8.3	8.1	7.7	5%
Tylenol Sinus Maximum Strength	8.5	**8.2**	**7.8**	33%
No Recommendation				17%

*Head congestion can be either nasal or sinus congestion or both.

• Indicates that this product was recommended by less than 1% of pharmacists surveyed.

Bold type indicates the highest rating.

Pharmacists Say...

PRODUCTS CONTAINING DECONGESTANTS may cause nervousness, dizziness, or sleeplessness.

IF YOU HAVE HEART DISEASE, high blood pressure, thyroid disease, diabetes, or prostate disease, contact your pharmacist or doctor before taking any product containing a decongestant.

IF YOU HAVE A HISTORY OF PEPTIC ULCERS, bleeding disorders, kidney disease, or asthma, contact your doctor before taking an over-the-counter anti-inflammatory medication such as aspirin, ibuprofen, naproxen, etc.

GENERIC EQUIVALENTS are available for these products. They are less expensive and just as effective as the name brands.

continued on next page

With chest congestion only:

EXPECTORANT

	Rated on a scale of 1 to 10			Percentage Of Pharmacists Who Most Often Recommend
	Most Effective	**Speed Of Relief**	**Desirable Duration Of Relief**	
Robitussin	**8.0**	**7.6**	**7.2**	**90%**
No Recommendation				10%

*With chest congestion **and** cough:*

EXPECTORANT, COUGH SUPPRESSANT COMBINATIONS

	Rated on a scale of 1 to 10			Percentage Of Pharmacists Who Most Often Recommend
	Most Effective	**Speed Of Relief**	**Desirable Duration Of Relief**	
Benylin Cough Suppressant Expectorant	8.2	7.9	7.4	3%
Cheracol D Cough Formula	8.0	7.8	7.4	3%
Robitussin DM	**8.5**	**8.1**	**7.5**	**89%**
Tolu-Sed DM	8.0	7.8	7.2	1%
No Recommendation				5%

*With chest congestion, cough, **and/or** head congestion:**

DECONGESTANT, EXPECTORANT, COUGH SUPPRESSANT COMBINATIONS

	Rated on a scale of 1 to 10			Percentage Of Pharmacists Who Most Often Recommend
	Most Effective	**Speed Of Relief**	**Desirable Duration Of Relief**	
Benylin Multi-Symptom	8.1	8.0	7.3	3%
Naldecon DX Adult Liquid	8.3	**8.2**	**7.7**	18%
Novahistine DMX	**8.4**	**8.2**	7.5	10%
Robitussin CF	8.3	8.1	7.5	**57%**
No Recommendation				12%

*Head congestion can be either nasal or sinus congestion or both.

• Indicates that this product was recommended by less than 1% of pharmacists surveyed.

Bold type indicates the highest rating.

COMBINATION PRODUCTS CONTAIN MANY INGREDIENTS. If you take such a product you may be taking more medication than you need and subjecting yourself to unnecessary side effects. Treat only the symptoms that you actually have.

PRODUCTS CONTAINING DECONGESTANTS may cause nervousness, dizziness, or sleeplessness.

IF YOU HAVE HEART DISEASE, high blood pressure, thyroid disease, diabetes, or prostate disease, contact your pharmacist or doctor before taking any product containing a decongestant.

DRY, NON-PHLEGM-PRODUCING COUGHS are best treated with a cough suppressant. Congested phlegm-producing coughs are best treated with an expectorant. However, if a congested cough is preventing you from sleeping at night, a cough suppressant and expectorant combination is recommended.

IF YOU HAVE A COUGH, you should increase your intake of fluids; six to eight glasses of plain water per day is recommended. However, if you have congestive heart failure or kidney problems, check with your doctor before increasing the amount of fluid you drink.

GENERIC EQUIVALENTS are available for these products. They are less expensive and just as effective as the name brands.

With sneezing, runny nose, watery eyes:

ANTIHISTAMINES

	Rated on a scale of 1 to 10			Percentage Of Pharmacists Who Most Often Recommend
	Most Effective	Ease Of Use	Speed Of Relief	
Benadryl Allergy	**8.6**	**7.6**	**8.1**	**58%**
Chlor-Trimeton Allergy	8.2	7.4	7.8	13%
Dimetapp Allergy Dye-Free Elixir	8.2	7.5	7.8	7%
Nolahist	7.1	6.9	7.4	•
No Recommendation				22%

• Indicates that this product was recommended by less than 1% of pharmacists surveyed.
Bold type indicates the highest rating.

Pharmacists Say...

IF YOUR CHILD HAS A HISTORY OF ASTHMA, chronic lung disease, or difficulty in urination, contact a doctor before giving your child any product containing an antihistamine.

ANTIHISTAMINES COMMONLY CAUSE DROWSINESS. However, in young children they may cause excitability.

SOME OF THESE PRODUCTS may contain alcohol or chemical dyes. Try to choose an alcohol-free and dye-free product for children.

GENERIC EQUIVALENTS are available for these products. They are less expensive and just as effective as the name brands.

With sneezing, runny nose, watery eyes, **and** *head congestion:**

ANTIHISTAMINE, DECONGESTANT COMBINATIONS

	Rated on a scale of 1 to 10			Percentage Of Pharmacists Who Most Often Recommend
	Most Effective	Desirable Duration Of Relief	Minimal Side Effects	
Benadryl Allergy Decongestant Liquid	8.4	7.4	6.8	9%
Dimetapp Cold & Allergy	**8.7**	**7.7**	**7.5**	**50%**
Triaminic Syrup Cold & Allergy	8.2	7.5	7.3	16%
No Recommendation				26%

*Head congestion can be either nasal or sinus congestion or both.
• Indicates that this product was recommended by less than 1% of pharmacists surveyed.
Bold type indicates the highest rating.

IF YOUR CHILD HAS A HISTORY OF ASTHMA, chronic lung disease, heart disease, high blood pressure, diabetes, thyroid disease, or difficulty in urination, contact a doctor before giving your child any product containing both an antihistamine and a decongestant.

GENERIC EQUIVALENTS are available for these products. They are less expensive and just as effective as the name-brands.

With head congestion* only:

DECONGESTANTS

| | Rated on a scale of 1 to 10 | | | Percentage Of Pharmacists Who Most Often Recommend |
	Most Effective	Ease Of Use	Speed Of Relief	
Dimetapp Decongestant Pediatric Drops	8.3	8.5	8.1	5%
PediaCare Infants' Decongestant	· 8.6	**8.6**	8.3	29%
Sudafed Children's Nasal Decongestant Liquid Medication	**8.8**	8.4	**8.4**	**59%**
Triaminic AM Non-Drowsy Decongestant	8.3	8.0	8.0	7%
No Recommendation				1%

*Head congestion can be either nasal or sinus congestion or both.
• Indicates that this product was recommended by less than 1% of pharmacists surveyed.
Bold type indicates the highest rating.

IF YOUR CHILD HAS A HISTORY OF HEART DISEASE, high blood pressure, diabetes, or thyroid disease, contact a doctor before giving your child any product containing a decongestant.

DECONGESTANTS may cause nervousness, dizziness, or sleeplessness.

THE ACTIVE INGREDIENT in these products is pseudoephedrine. This ingredient is available in generic products, which cost less and are just as effective as name brands.

DECONGESTANTS ARE CONSIDERED NONSEDATING because they don't contain antihistamines.

continued on next page

ANTIHISTAMINE, DECONGESTANT, COUGH SUPPRESSANT COMBINATIONS

| | *Rated on a scale of 1 to 10* | | | Percentage Of |
	Most Effective	Desirable Duration Of Relief	Speed Of Relief	Pharmacists Who Most Often Recommend
PediaCare NightRest Cough-Cold	**8.5**	**7.8**	**8.0**	**27%**
Triaminic Triaminicol Cold & Cough	8.3	7.6	**8.0**	**27%**
Triaminic Night Time Maximum Strength	8.2	7.7	7.9	11%
Tylenol** Children's Cold Multi Symptom Plus Cough	8.3	7.6	**8.0**	15%
Vicks 44m Pediatric Cough & Cold Relief	8.1	7.4	7.9	3%
Vicks Nyquil Children's Cold/Cough Relief	8.0	7.5	7.7	4%
No Recommendation				13%

* Head congestion can be either nasal or sinus congestion or both.

** This product also contains a pain reliever, which may not be necessary to treat the above symptoms.

Bold type indicates the highest rating.

Pharmacists Say..

COMBINATION PRODUCTS CONTAIN MANY INGREDIENTS. If you give your children such a product you may be giving them more medication than they need and subjecting them to unnecessary side effects. Treat only the symptoms that they actually have.

IF YOUR CHILD HAS A HISTORY OF ASTHMA, chronic lung disease, heart disease, high blood pressure, diabetes, thyroid disease, or difficulty in urination, contact a doctor before giving your child any product containing both an antihistamine and a decongestant.

GENERIC EQUIVALENTS are available for these products. They are less expensive and just as effective as the name brands.

With chest congestion only:

EXPECTORANT

| | Rated on a scale of 1 to 10 | | | Percentage Of Pharmacists Who Most Often Recommend |
	Most Effective	Desirable Duration Of Relief	Minimal Side Effects	
Robitussin	**8.2**	**7.6**	**8.5**	**90%**
No Recommendation				10%

With chest congestion **and** cough:

EXPECTORANT, COUGH SUPPRESSANT COMBINATIONS

| | Rated on a scale of 1 to 10 | | | Percentage Of Pharmacists Who Most Often Recommend |
	Most Effective	Desirable Duration Of Relief	Speed Of Relief	
Benylin Cough Suppressant Expectorant	8.2	7.5	7.9	5%
Cheracol D Cough Formula	8.2	7.5	8.1	4%
Robitussin DM	**8.6**	**7.7**	**8.6**	**80%**
Vicks 44e Pediatric Cough & Chest Congestion Relief	8.0	7.5	7.8	6%
No Recommendation				6%

With chest congestion, cough, **and/or** head congestion:*

DECONGESTANT, EXPECTORANT, COUGH SUPPRESSANT COMBINATIONS

| | Rated on a scale of 1 to 10 | | | Percentage Of Pharmacists Who Most Often Recommend |
	Most Effective	Desirable Duration Of Relief	Speed Of Relief	
Benylin Multi-Symptom	8.2	7.5	7.9	7%
Dorcol Children's Cough Syrup	8.0	7.3	7.9	8%
Naldecon DX Children's Syrup	**8.6**	**7.8**	**8.2**	32%
Robitussin Pediatric	8.3	7.7	8.1	**36%**
Triaminic** Sore Throat, Throat Pain & Cough	7.7	7.4	7.8	6%
No Recommendation				12%

*Head congestion can be either nasal or sinus congestion or both.

**This product also contains a pain reliever, which may not be necessary to treat the above symptoms.

Bold type indicates the highest rating.

continued on next page

39

COMBINATION PRODUCTS CONTAIN MANY INGREDIENTS. If you give your child such a product you may be giving them more medication than they need and subjecting them to unnecessary side effects. Treat only the symptoms that they actually have.

IF YOUR CHILD HAS A HISTORY OF HEART DISEASE, high blood pressure, diabetes, or thyroid disease, contact a doctor before giving your child any product containing a decongestant.

DRY, NON-PHLEGM-PRODUCING COUGHS are best treated with a cough suppressant. Congested phlegm-producing coughs are best treated with an expectorant. However, if a congested cough is preventing your child from sleeping at night, a cough suppressant and expectorant combination is recommended.

INCREASING FLUID INTAKE AND USING A HUMIDIFIER will also help to relieve your child's chest congestion.

GENERIC EQUIVALENTS are available for these products. They are less expensive and just as effective as the name brands.

If you have a high fever, severe headache, stiff neck, confusion, lethargy, a cough that produces green or yellow phlegm, or shortness of breath, consult your doctor immediately. Furthermore, if you don't feel better after four to seven days, or if you experience side effects from over-the-counter medications, you should see your doctor.

Cold sores

The majority of cold sores are due to a recurrence of a herpes infection that was acquired during childhood. Sunlight, stress, illness, and hormonal changes allow the virus to become active again in the form of ulcers.

SYMPTOMS: *Ulcers or sores on the inside of the mouth • Crusty sores on the lips*

| | *Rated on a scale of 1 to 10* | | | Percentage Of Pharmacists Who Most Often Recommend |
	Most Effective	Speed Of Relief	Ease Of Use	
Anbesol Maximum Strength	7.2	**7.7**	8.3	5%
Blistex Medicated Lip Ointment	6.7	6.6	8.4	1%
Blistex Lip Medex	6.7	6.7	8.4	2%
Campho-phenique Original Cold Sore Gel	7.2	7.1	8.2	7%
Carmex Lip Balm	7.3	7.1	**8.5**	26%
Orabase-B With Benzocaine	7.4	7.5	7.9	10%
Orajel Mouth-Aid	7.2	7.6	8.3	3%
Tanac No Sting	7.0	7.2	7.8	4%
Zilactin Medicated Gel	**7.8**	7.6	8.4	**30%**
No Recommendation				12%

Bold type indicates the highest rating.

Pharmacists Say...

COLD SORES HEAL ON THEIR OWN. These products keep the cold sore moisturized, preventing the sore from cracking and spreading to surrounding areas.

USING BLISTEX OR CARMEX, even if you don't have a cold sore, will help to prevent cold sores.

GELS MAY PROVIDE longer-lasting relief than liquids, because they don't rinse away as easily.

AFTER APPLYING ANY OF THESE PRODUCTS, try to wait at least a half hour before eating or drinking to make sure that the medication isn't washed away, which will decrease its effectiveness.

See Your Doctor...

If cold sores don't clear up after ten to fourteen days, or recur frequently, contact your doctor.

See also *Canker Sores*

Congestion: Chest

Chest congestion is a symptom of bronchitis, which is an inflammation of the bronchial tubes. Bronchitis is frequently caused by the same viruses that cause colds. Chest congestion is also a symptom frequently associated with asthma and chronic pulmonary disease, as well as a condition prevalent among cigarette smokers. You can obtain relief by using a humidifier or vaporizer to add moisture to the air. If you have chest congestion that is due to colds, refer to the charts under colds on page 34.

SYMPTOMS: *Congestion, with or without a cough*

See Your Doctor...

In general, patients, with a history of heart or lung disease need to consult their doctor at the onset of chest congestion. Chest congestion associated with shortness of breath, high fevers, excessive phlegm (mucus), chest pain, and severe fatigue or weakness, should be evaluated by a doctor. Furthermore, if you don't feel better after four to seven days, or if you experience side effects from over-the-counter medications, you should contact your doctor.

See also *Colds; Coughs*

Congestion: Head

Head congestion refers to nasal or sinus congestion or both. The most common causes of head congestion are allergies, such as hayfever, or colds. If your head congestion is due to allergies, refer to the charts and tips on pages 6–7. If your head congestion is due to colds, refer to the charts and tips on pages 30–33. In addition, you can obtain relief by using a humidifier or vaporizer to add moisture to the air, or by drinking plenty of fluids. The following decongestant and saline sprays are used to alleviate head congestion in both allergies and colds.

SYMPTOMS: *Clogged or stuffy nose*

DECONGESTANT NASAL SPRAYS (*For adults only. Do not administer to children*)

| | Rated on a scale of 1 to 10 | | | Percentage Of Pharmacists Who Most Often Recommend |
	Minimal Side Effects	Most Effective	Speed Of Relief	
Afrin 12 Hour Nasal Spray	**7.3**	**8.9**	**9.0**	**88%**
Dristan 12-Hour Nasal Spray	7.1	8.6	8.7	•
Duration 12 Hour Spray	7.1	8.6	8.8	1%
No Recommendation				11%

SALINE SPRAYS

| | Rated on a scale of 1 to 10 | | | Percentage Of Pharmacists Who Most Often Recommend |
	Minimal Side Effects	Most Effective	Speed Of Relief	
Afrin Saline Mist	9.4	**7.9**	8.0	4%
Ayr Non-Medicated Saline Nasal	9.4	7.8	**8.1**	10%
NaSal Saline Moisturizer	**9.5**	**7.9**	**8.1**	5%
Ocean	**9.5**	**7.9**	**8.1**	77%
No Recommendation				4%

• Indicates that this product was recommended by less than 1% of pharmacists surveyed.

Bold type indicates the highest rating.

continued on next page

See also *Allergies; Colds*

DECONGESTANT NASAL SPRAYS shouldn't be used for more than three to four days. Using them for longer periods can worsen your nasal congestion. Additionally, these medications are potentially habit forming.

TO PREVENT THE SPREAD OF GERMS, only one person should use a bottle of nasal spray. When the congestion is better, throw away the spray bottle. It should not be used again, because it may have been contaminated.

SALINE SPRAYS MAY NOT PROVIDE RELIEF QUITE AS QUICKLY AS DECONGESTANT SPRAYS, but they can be used as often as necessary, and they are effective and safe. For children, you may need a nasal syringe to remove the mucus.

GENERIC EQUIVALENTS are available for these products. They are less expensive and just as effective as the name brands.

If your congestion doesn't improve after four to seven days and is accompanied by fever or headache, contact your doctor.

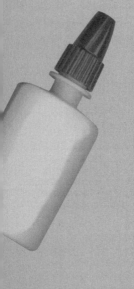

Constipation

Constipation is best described as a decrease in your usual bowel function. Common causes include decreased fiber in your diet, a decrease in your amount of fluid intake, a lack of physical activity, certain medications, and travel. Additionally, overuse of laxatives can be a cause of recurrent constipation. Before you take medication for constipation, try to promote regularity by exercising, increasing your dietary fiber intake, and drinking more water. The over-the-counter products listed below are meant for temporary relief of constipation. If you have persistent constipation, you should see your doctor.

SYMPTOMS: *Infrequent bowel movements*
• Hard, dry movements

For Adults

STOOL SOFTENERS AND LUBRICANTS

| | Rated on a scale of 1 to 10 | | | Percentage Of Pharmacists Who Most Often Recommend |
	Most Effective	Speed Of Relief	Minimal Side Effects	
Colace	**8.8**	6.9	**9.0**	**87%**
Kondremul	7.9	**7.2**	7.7	•
Surfak Stool Softener	8.7	6.8	8.8	11%
No Recommendation				2%

• *Indicates that this product was recommended by less than 1% of pharmacists surveyed.*
Bold type indicates the highest rating.

Pharmacists Say...

STOOL SOFTENERS ARE A GOOD CHOICE for chronic constipation that does not respond to increased exercise, water, and fiber. However, if you need immediate relief, products containing mineral oil such as Kondremul, will work more quickly than products containing docusate, such as Colace and Surfak.

STOOL SOFTENERS CONTAINING DOCUSATE should be taken with plenty of water. Additionally, keep in mind that these products will need several days to work.

GENERIC EQUIVALENTS are available for these products. They are less expensive and just as effective as the name brands.

continued on next page

	Rated on a scale of 1 to 10			Percentage Of Pharmacists Who Most Often Recommend
	Most Effective	**Speed Of Relief**	**Minimal Side Effects**	
Correctol Bisacodyl Stimulant Laxative	8.2	7.6	7.1	9%
Doxidan	8.0	7.4	**7.5**	8%
Dulcolax Tablets	**9.0**	8.3	7.3	**56%**
Ex-Lax Regular Strength Laxative Pills	8.2	7.8	6.9	3%
Feen-A-Mint Bisacodyl Stimulant Laxative	8.0	7.6	6.8	•
Fleet Phospho-Soda Buffered Saline Oral Laxative	**9.0**	**8.8**	6.7	3%
Fletcher's Castoria	7.8	7.5	7.1	•
Haley's M-O Lubricant Laxative	7.9	7.5	6.9	1%
Nature's Remedy	7.9	7.6	7.4	1%
Philip's Milk Of Magnesia Laxative/Antacid	7.9	7.5	7.1	16%
No Recommendation				4%

• Indicates that this product was recommended by less than 1% of pharmacists surveyed.

Bold type indicates the highest rating.

Pharmacists Say...

STIMULANT LAXATIVES should be used only occasionally. Excessive use can cause severe cramping, diarrhea, vomiting, and loss of important body chemicals such as potassium. Stool softeners or fiber-based laxatives are better choices for frequent use.

GENERIC EQUIVALENTS are available for these products. They are less expensive and just as effective as the name brands.

| | Rated on a scale of 1 to 10 | | | Percentage Of Pharmacists Who Most Often Recommend |
	Most Effective	Speed Of Relief	Minimal Side Effects	
Citrucel Fiber Therapy for Regularity	**8.4**	**6.9**	**8.2**	32%
Fiberall Premium Psyllium Fiber	8.1	6.5	7.8	•
FiberCon	8.1	6.6	8.0	18%
Konsyl Psyllium Hydrophilic Mucilloid	8.2	6.7	7.8	1%
Metamucil Smooth Texture	8.3	6.7	8.0	**38%**
Perdiem Fiber	8.3	6.8	7.8	7%
No Recommendation				4%

• Indicates that this product was recommended by less than 1% of pharmacists surveyed.
Bold type indicates the highest rating.

Pharmacists Say...

FIBER SUPPLEMENTS are an excellent choice for chronic constipation, though they need to be used on a regular basis. It's important to drink at least eight glasses of water per day while taking fiber supplements, to avoid potential obstruction in the gastrointestinal tract.

FIBER SUPPLEMENTS can affect the absorption of some prescription medications. If you're taking other medications, check with your doctor or pharmacist before using these products.

YOU MIGHT FIND the fiber powders easier to drink if they're mixed with juice.

FIBER PRODUCTS can cause increased gas production, although this may be less of a problem with Citrucel.

BEFORE YOU TAKE MEDICATION for constipation, try exercising, increasing your dietary fiber by eating high-fiber foods, and drinking more water to promote regularity.

GENERIC EQUIVALENTS are available for these products. They are less expensive and just as effective as the name brands.

continued on next page

| | Rated on a scale of 1 to 10 | | | Percentage Of |
	Most Effective	Speed Of Relief	Ease Of Use	Pharmacists Who Most Often Recommend
Dulcolax Suppositories	**9.2**	8.8	7.7	**54%**
Fleet Glycerin Suppositories	8.1	8.2	7.6	22%
Fleet Ready-to-Use Enema	**9.2**	**9.2**	6.7	16%
Senokot Suppositories	8.4	8.2	**8.0**	1%
No Recommendation				7%

Bold type indicates the highest rating.

Pharmacists Say...

SUPPOSITORIES are easier to insert if you dampen them with water first.

IF YOU'RE RELUCTANT TO USE AN ENEMA, try glycerin suppositories. They are the least harsh and work quickly.

FOR A HARD, DRY STOOL, suppositories will not be as effective as enemas.

GENERIC EQUIVALENTS are available for these products. They are less expensive and just as effective as the name brands.

For Children

STOOL SOFTENERS/LUBRICANTS

| | Rated on a scale of 1 to 10 | | | Percentage Of |
	Most Effective	Speed Of Relief	Desirable Duration Of Relief	Pharmacists Who Most Often Recommend
Agoral Stimulant Laxative	7.9	**7.5**	7.6	10%
Colace Liquid	**8.5**	7.2	**7.8**	**77%**
No Recommendation				12%

Bold type indicates the highest rating.

STIMULANTS

| | Rated on a scale of 1 to 10 | | | Percentage Of Pharmacists Who Most Often Recommend |
	Most Effective	Speed Of Relief	Desirable Duration Of Relief	
Dulcolax Tablet	8.5	7.8	7.5	5%
Fleet Phospho-Soda Buffered Saline Oral Laxative	**8.6**	**8.6**	7.5	4%
Fletcher's Cherry The Children's Laxative	8.3	7.9	7.6	**40%**
Philip's Milk Of Magnesia Laxative/Antacid	7.8	7.5	7.4	19%
Senokot Children's Syrup	8.2	7.8	**7.7**	16%
No Recommendation				16%

SUPPOSITORIES

| | Rated on a scale of 1 to 10 | | | Percentage Of Pharmacists Who Most Often Recommend |
	Most Effective	Speed Of Relief	Desirable Duration Of Relief	
Dulcolax Suppositories	**8.9**	**8.7**	**8.0**	5%
Fleet Glycerin Suppositories (Child Size)	8.6	8.5	**8.0**	**90%**
No Recommendation				5%

Bold type indicates the highest rating.

Pharmacists Say...

PHARMACISTS RECOMMEND AGAINST TREATING CONSTIPA-
TION IN CHILDREN WITHOUT CONSULTING A DOCTOR.

FRUIT JUICES (such as prune, apple, or pear juice) may be the
only treatment required.

See Your Doctor...

*If your constipation is associated with abdominal pain,
nausea, vomiting, or blood in the stools, contact your doctor immediately. Also you should see your doctor if you
have noticed a change in bowel habits that persist for
more than two weeks.*

Corns and Calluses

Corns and calluses are areas of thickened skin caused by constant friction and pressure. The skin beneath the thickened area is usually tender and painful. Corns are small and form on the toes and feet; calluses are larger and form on the bottom of the foot. (Calluses can also occur on your hands if you regularly perform heavy manual labor.) To prevent corns and calluses on your feet, be sure to wear comfortable, loose-fitting shoes. If you have corns or calluses, you can stop the pain by removing the dead skin with a pumice stone, by keeping your feet moisturized, and by applying a special cushion that keeps direct pressure off the area.

SYMPTOMS: *Corn—small overgrowth of skin sensitive to pressure. Callus—rough, hard patch of skin*

	Rated on a scale of 1 to 10			Percentage Of Pharmacists Who Most Often Recommend
	Most Effective	**Speed Of Relief**	**Ease Of Use**	
Dr. Scholl's Advanced Pain Relief Callus Removers	**8.0**	6.9	8.0	5%
Dr. Scholl's Advanced Pain Relief Corn Removers	**8.0**	6.9	8.0	11%
Dr. Scholl's Liquid Corn/Callus Remover	7.8	6.8	7.1	22%
Dr. Scholl's One Step Callus Removers	**8.0**	**7.0**	**8.2**	7%
Dr. Scholl's One Step Corn Removers	**8.0**	6.9	8.1	7%
Dr. Scholl's Soft Corn Removers	7.7	6.8	7.8	5%
Dr. Scholl's Wrap-Around Corn Removers	7.8	6.9	7.8	4%
Freezone Corn and Callus Remover	7.8	6.8	7.1	15%
Off-Ezy Corn and Callus Remover Kit	7.5	6.6	6.8	0%
No Recommendation				**25%**

• *Indicates that this product was recommended by less than 1% of pharmacists surveyed.*

Bold type indicates the highest rating.

BEFORE APPLYING MEDICATION to a corn or callus, you might want to apply a thin coat of Vaseline to the normal skin around the area. This protects the normal skin from the "burning" effect of the medication.

Patients with diabetes or other vascular problems should consult their doctor if they experience any type of foot problem. If you have corns or calluses that don't respond to over-the-counter medications, or if irritation occurs as a result of these products, contact your doctor.

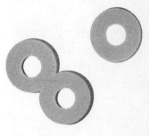

Coughs

Coughing is the body's response to irritation in the respiratory tract. The most common causes include infections such as colds, bronchitis, and pneumonia. Chronic coughing may be caused by asthma, sinus conditions, cigarette smoking, certain medications, or exposure to environmental irritants such as dust. The following over-the-counter products should not be taken for chronic coughs unless you're directed to do so by your doctor.

SYMPTOMS: *Coughing*

For Adults

With a cough only:

COUGH SUPPRESSANTS

| | Rated on a scale of 1 to 10 | | | Percentage Of Pharmacists Who Most Often Recommend |
	Most Effective	Speed Of Relief	Desirable Duration Of Relief	
Benylin Adult Formula	8.0	7.8	7.3	14%
Drixoral Cough Liquid Caps	8.0	7.6	7.2	9%
Pertussin DM Extra Strength Cough Relief	7.7	7.8	6.8	3%
Robitussin Maximum Strength Cough	**8.3**	**8.0**	**7.6**	**51%**
No Recommendation				23%

*With a cough **and** chest congestion:*

EXPECTORANT, COUGH SUPPRESSANT COMBINATIONS

| | Rated on a scale of 1 to 10 | | | Percentage Of Pharmacists Who Most Often Recommend |
	Most Effective	Speed Of Relief	Desirable Duration Of Relief	
Benylin Cough Suppressant Expectorant	8.2	7.9	7.4	3%
Cheracol D Cough Formula	8.0	7.8	7.4	3%
Robitussin DM	**8.5**	**8.1**	**7.5**	**89%**
Tolu-Sed DM	8.0	7.8	7.2	1%
No Recommendation				5%

Bold type indicates the highest rating.

See also *Colds; Congestion: Chest*

*With a cough, chest congestion, **and/or** head congestion:**

DECONGESTANT, EXPECTORANT, COUGH SUPPRESSANT COMBINATIONS

| | Rated on a scale of 1 to 10 | | | Percentage Of Pharmacists Who Most Often Recommend |
	Most Effective	Speed Of Relief	Desirable Duration Of Relief	
Benylin Multi-Symptom	8.1	8.0	7.3	3%
Naldecon DX Adult Liquid	8.3	**8.2**	**7.7**	18%
Novahistine DMX	**8.4**	**8.2**	7.5	10%
Robitussin CF	8.3	8.1	7.5	**57%**
No Recommendation				12%

*Head congestion can be either nasal or sinus congestion or both.
Bold type indicates the highest rating.

Pharmacists Say...

DRY, NON-PHLEGM-PRODUCING COUGHS are best treated with a cough suppressant. Congested phlegm-producing coughs are best treated with an expectorant. However, if a congested cough is preventing you from sleeping at night, a cough suppressant and expectorant combination is recommended.

PRODUCTS CONTAINING DECONGESTANTS may cause nervousness, dizziness, or sleeplessness.

IF YOU HAVE HEART DISEASE, high blood pressure, thyroid disease, diabetes, or prostate disease, contact your pharmacist or doctor before taking any product containing a decongestant.

IF YOU HAVE A COUGH, you should increase your intake of fluids; six to eight glasses of plain water per day is recommended. However, if you have congestive heart failure or kidney problems, check with your doctor before increasing the amount of fluid you drink.

COMBINATION PRODUCTS CONTAIN MANY INGREDIENTS. If you take such a product you may be taking more medication than you need and subjecting yourself to unnecessary side effects. Treat only the symptoms that you actually have.

GENERIC EQUIVALENTS are available for these products. They are less expensive and just as effective as the name brands.

continued on next page

With all coughs, with or without symptoms:

COUGH DROPS, LOZENGES

	Rated on a scale of 1 to 10			Percentage Of Pharmacists Who Most Often Recommend
	Most Effective	**Speed Of Relief**	**Desirable Duration Of Relief**	
Cough-X	**7.8**	**8.0**	**7.0**	9%
Hold DM	**7.8**	7.7	6.9	16%
Sucrets 4-Hour Cough Suppressant	**7.8**	7.7	6.8	18%
No Recommendation				**57%**

Bold type indicates the highest rating.

IF YOU HAVE A SORE THROAT AS WELL AS A COUGH, you might try lozenges that contain benzocaine, a mild anesthetic that numbs throat pain.

SUGAR-FREE HARD CANDY soothes a cough as well as medicated lozenges do.

For Children

With a cough only:

COUGH SUPPRESSANTS

	Rated on a scale of 1 to 10			Percentage Of Pharmacists Who Most Often Recommend
	Most Effective	**Desirable Duration Of Relief**	**Speed Of Relief**	
Benylin Pediatric	8.0	7.2	7.8	7%
Delsym 12 Hour Cough Relief Cough Formula	**8.7**	**8.8**	7.9	**45%**
Robitussin Pediatric Cough	8.3	7.5	**8.0**	39%
No Recommendation				10%

Bold type indicates the highest rating.

With a cough **and** *head congestion:**

ANTIHISTAMINE, DECONGESTANT, COUGH SUPPRESSANT COMBINATIONS

	Rated on a scale of 1 to 10			Percentage Of Pharmacists Who Most Often Recommend
	Most Effective	**Desirable Duration Of Relief**	**Speed Of Relief**	
PediaCare NightRest Cough-Cold	**8.5**	**7.8**	**8.0**	**27%**
Triaminic Triaminicol Cold & Cough	8.3	7.6	**8.0**	**27%**
Triaminic Night Time Maximum Strength	8.2	7.7	7.9	11%
Tylenol** Children's Cold Multi Symptom Plus Cough	8.3	7.6	**8.0**	15%
Vicks 44m Pediatric Cough & Cold Relief	8.1	7.4	7.9	3%
Vicks Nyquil Children's Cold/Cough Relief	8.0	7.5	7.7	4%
No Recommendation				13%

*Head congestion can be either nasal or sinus congestion or both.

**This product also contains a pain reliever, which may not be necessary to treat the above symptoms.

Bold type indicates the highest rating.

With a cough **and** *chest congestion:*

EXPECTORANT, COUGH SUPPRESSANT

	Rated on a scale of 1 to 10			Percentage Of Pharmacists Who Most Often Recommend
	Most Effective	**Desirable Duration Of Relief**	**Speed Of Relief**	
Benylin Cough Suppressant Expectorant	8.2	7.5	7.9	5%
Cheracol D Cough Formula	8.2	7.5	8.1	4%
Robitussin DM	**8.6**	**7.7**	**8.6**	**80%**
Vicks 44e Pediatric Cough & Chest Congestion Relief	8.0	7.5	7.8	6%
No Recommendation				6%

Bold type indicates the highest rating.

*With a cough, chest congestion, **and** head congestion:**

DECONGESTANT, EXPECTORANT, COUGH SUPPRESSANT COMBINATIONS

	Rated on a scale of 1 to 10			Percentage Of Pharmacists Who Most Often Recommend
	Most Effective	**Desirable Duration Of Relief**	**Speed Of Relief**	
Benylin Multi-Symptom	8.2	7.5	7.9	7%
Dorcol Children's Cough Syrup	8.0	7.3	7.9	8%
Naldecon DX Children's Syrup	**8.6**	**7.8**	**8.2**	32%
Robitussin Pediatric	8.3	7.7	8.1	**36%**
Triaminic** Sore Throat, Throat Pain & Cough	7.7	7.4	7.8	6%
No Recommendation				12%

Head congestion can be either nasal or sinus congestion or both.
**This product also contains a pain reliever, which may not be necessary to treat the above symptoms.*
Bold type indicates the highest rating.

Pharmacists Say...

DRY, NON-PHLEGM-PRODUCING COUGHS are best treated with a cough suppressant. Congested phlegm-producing coughs are best treated with an expectorant. However, if a congested cough is preventing your child from sleeping at night, a cough suppressant and expectorant combination is recommended.

INCREASING FLUID INTAKE AND USING A HUMIDIFIER will also help to relieve your child's chest congestion.

COMBINATION PRODUCTS CONTAIN MANY INGREDIENTS. If you give your children such a product you may be giving them more medication than they need and subjecting them to unnecessary side effects. Treat only the symptoms that they actually have.

IF YOUR CHILD HAS A HISTORY OF ASTHMA, chronic lung disease, or difficulty in urination contact a doctor before giving your child any product containing an antihistamine. Likewise, if your child has a history of heart disease, high blood pressure, or thyroid disease contact a doctor before giving your child any product containing a decongestant.

GENERIC EQUIVALENTS are available for these products. They are less expensive and just as effective as the name brands.

With all coughs, with or without symptoms:

COUGH DROPS, LOZENGES

	Rated on a scale of 1 to 10			Percentage Of Pharmacists Who Most Often Recommend
	Most Effective	**Desirable Duration Of Relief**	**Speed Of Relief**	
Hold DM	**7.8**	**7.3**	**7.6**	29%
No Recommendation				**72%**

Bold type indicates the highest rating.

Pharmacists Say...

BECAUSE OF THE RISK OF CHOKING, be very careful when giving lozenges to children. Do not let children run, play, or lie down with a lozenge in their mouth.

CHILDREN HAVE A TENDENCY TO SWALLOW COUGH DROPS and lozenges, which lessens their effectiveness at treating the sore throat.

BE SURE THAT THE CHILD doesn't use lozenges or sprays that contain an anesthetic within an hour or two before eating; a numb throat makes it easier for a child to choke on food.

See Your Doctor...

A persistent cough may be a sign of a serious condition. If your cough lasts for more than one week, tends to recur, or is accompanied by a fever, rash, persistent headache, difficulty breathing, chest pain, or excessive phlegm (mucus), consult your doctor.

Cuts and Scrapes

Slight bleeding from a cut or scrape will usually stop on its own; if it doesn't, apply pressure to the area by pressing a sterile gauze pad firmly over the wound. Cuts and scrapes should always be cleaned with antibacterial soap and water; topical antibiotics can be applied to prevent infection and promote quicker healing. Cuts heal best when they're covered, so be sure to apply a bandage after cleaning the wound.

SYMPTOMS: *Red or broken skin • Minor bleeding*

| | Rated on a scale of 1 to 10 | | | Percentage Of Pharmacists Who Most Often Recommend |
	Most Effective	Speed Of Relief	Desirable Duration Of Relief	
Baciguent	7.6	7.3	7.6	2%
Bactine First Aid Antiseptic	7.5	7.9	7.3	1%
Betadine Solution	8.2	7.5	7.3	2%
Campho-phenique Pain Relieving Antiseptic	7.1	7.5	7.2	1%
Neosporin Original	8.9	7.9	8.1	57%
Neosporin Plus Maximum Strength	**9.0**	**8.6**	**8.3**	**24%**
Polysporin First Aid Antibiotic	8.5	7.8	8.1	8%
No Recommendation				6%

Bold type indicates the highest rating.

Pharmacists Say...

IF YOU'RE ALLERGIC TO NEOMYCIN (the active ingredient in Neosporin), try using Polysporin or Baciguent or their generic equivalents.

BE CAREFUL WHEN USING BETADINE, as it stains clothing.

THESE PRODUCTS ARE MOST EFFECTIVE in preventing an infection and less effective in curing one. The wound should be cleaned and treated with these medications as soon as possible so that infection doesn't occur.

GENERIC EQUIVALENTS are available for these products. They are less expensive and just as effective as the name brands.

If you have been cut on your face or have a cut that is deep or irregular and does not stop bleeding after applying pressure, see your doctor. Any patient with a deep cut should make sure their tetanus immunization is up to date. Furthermore, if you develop a fever, redness or pus at the site of the wound, contact your doctor, because this could indicate an infection.

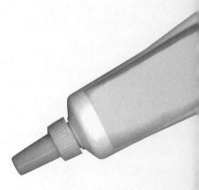

Dandruff

The white flakes associated with dandruff are caused by accelerated growth of skin cells on the scalp. This process occurs with seborrhea or psoriasis. Dandruff isn't a health-threatening ailment.

SYMPTOMS: *White flakes on the scalp that may fall onto the shoulders • Itchy or scaly scalp*

	Rated on a scale of 1 to 10			Percentage Of Pharmacists Who Most Often Recommend
	Most Effective	**Speed Of Relief**	**Ease Of Use**	
Denorex Medicated Shampoo	7.9	7.6	8.4	5%
Head & Shoulders Dandruff Shampoo	7.6	7.4	8.8	19%
Ionil	7.3	7.1	8.1	1%
Ionil T Plus	7.7	7.3	8.0	1%
Neutrogena Therapeutic T/Gel Shampoo	**8.4**	**7.8**	8.4	30%
Sebulex Medicated Dandruff Shampoo	8.0	7.4	8.4	4%
Sebutone Tar Shampoo	8.1	7.3	8.2	3%
Selsun Blue Dandruff Shampoo Medicated Treatment	8.1	7.6	**8.9**	**31%**
Tegrin Dandruff Shampoo	7.7	7.4	8.4	•
X-Seb	7.7	7.2	8.2	•
X-Seb T Pearl	8.2	7.3	8.0	1%
No Recommendation				5%

• Indicates that this product was recommended by less than 1% of pharmacists surveyed.
Bold type indicates the highest rating.

Pharmacists Say...

YOU MAY NEED TO TREAT DANDRUFF for several weeks before you begin to see an improvement. Your best bet is to start with mild products such as Selsun Blue or Head & Shoulders before trying other products with harsher ingredients. This way you can find the mildest product that works well for you, though it may not be the first one you try.

TAR-BASED SHAMPOOS should be used only to treat stubborn problems that don't respond to other products. These shampoos are not recommended for daily use and should be alternated with non-tar-based products.

FOR MILD CASES OF DANDRUFF, an inexpensive dandruff shampoo will give the same results as the more expensive brands.

See Your Doctor...

If the dandruff doesn't improve after four weeks of using over-the-counter medications, contact your doctor.

Diaper Rash

Diaper rash is caused by extended contact with irritating elements, such as moisture, detergent, or bowel movements. To avoid diaper rash, change the baby's diapers as quickly as possible after soiling, and keep the baby's bottom as clean as possible. Superabsorbent disposable diapers are very effective in keeping moisture away from the baby's skin. If you use cloth diapers, be sure that all detergent has been completely rinsed from the diapers before using them. Exposure to air will help diaper rash clear quickly, so if it's possible let the baby spend some time without diapers or with the diaper unfastened. (For example, the baby can take a nap while lying on an opened, unfastened diaper.)

SYMPTOMS: *Red, moist spots on area covered by diapers*

	Rated on a scale of 1 to 10			Percentage Of Pharmacists Who Most Often Recommend
	Most Effective	**Minimal Side Effects**	**Ease Of Use**	
A and D Medicated Diaper Rash Ointment With Zinc Oxide	7.6	**8.8**	**8.8**	24%
Desitin Diaper Rash Ointment	**7.9**	**8.8**	8.4	**41%**
Desitin Cornstarch Baby Powder	7.8	8.7	8.7	5%
Diaparene Cornstarch Baby Powder	6.8	8.2	8.2	1%
Diaparene Diaper Rash Ointment	7.7	8.6	8.6	3%
Johnson's Diaper Rash Ointment	7.3	8.4	8.2	4%
No Recommendation				23%

Bold type indicates the highest rating.

Pharmacists Say...

THESE PRODUCTS ARE GOOD for preventing a rash or clearing a minor irritation, but they may make a yeast infection worse by keeping in moisture.

TO PREVENT DIAPER RASH, apply ointment to the diaper area, especially at bedtime, since exposure to wet diapers may be prolonged overnight.

MAKE SURE THAT THE CHILD doesn't inhale any powder when you're applying it to the diaper area.

See Your Doctor...

If the condition worsens or does not improve with the recommendations outlined above, contact your doctor.

Dermatitis

Dermatitis is a term that encompasses a variety of ailments that cause an inflammation of the skin. One of the most common types, "contact dermatitis," is a result of touching a substance that causes a reaction, such as poison ivy or certain metals in jewelry or watchbands. Another kind of dermatitis can occur from frequent exposure to household detergents or other chemicals. Dermatitis causes itching, but scratching an affected area can make it worse. If you have dermatitis on your hands, wear cotton gloves under rubber gloves to prevent further irritation while you wash dishes or use household chemicals. Also, try to avoid using dyed or scented soaps and tissues, as they may aggravate your condition.

SYMPTOMS: *Patches of red, itchy skin*
• Tiny blisters on the affected area

| | Rated on a scale of 1 to 10 | | | Percentage Of Pharmacists Who Most Often Recommend |
	Most Effective	Speed Of Relief	Desirable Duration Of Relief	
Cortaid Maximum Strength	**8.6**	**8.1**	7.8	**50%**
Corticaine Maximum Strength	8.5	8.0	**7.9**	4%
Cortizone-10	**8.6**	8.0	7.8	33%
Kericort 10	8.3	7.8	7.6	•
Lanacort 10	8.3	7.9	7.7	2%
No Recommendation				11%

• Indicates that this product was recommended by less than 1% of pharmacists surveyed.
Bold type indicates the highest rating.

Pharmacists Say...

THESE PRODUCTS ARE USUALLY EFFECTIVE ONLY on minor skin irritations. When using these products, you should use a moisturizer regularly to increase the penetration of hydrocortisone and reduce itching.

GENERIC HYDROCORTISONE is less expensive and just as effective as the name-brand products.

HYDROCORTISONE should not be used on skin that is broken or bleeding.

THESE PRODUCTS MUST BE USED for three to four days before they'll achieve the best results.

See Your Doctor...

If the condition worsens, doesn't improve, or recurs after taking over-the-counter medication, contact your doctor.

See also *Dry Skin*

Diarrhea

Diarrhea can be caused by a number of factors, including bacteria, viruses, stress, change of diet, and even certain medicines. If you have diarrhea, be sure that you drink plenty of liquids so that you don't become dehydrated. You should also avoid foods that will irritate your condition, such as dairy products and fried or greasy foods. Drink clear liquids for a few days and stick to a bland diet such as toast, bananas, and cereal.

SYMPTOMS: *Loose, watery stools • Abdominal cramps • Frequent need to move bowels*

	Rated on a scale of 1 to 10			Percentage Of Pharmacists Who Most Often Recommend
	Most Effective	Speed Of Relief	Desirable Duration Of Relief	
Donnagel	7.6	7.4	7.2	2%
Equalactin Chew Tablets	6.9	6.4	6.5	1%
Imodium A-D	**9.3**	**8.8**	**8.8**	**90%**
Kaopectate	7.6	7.3	7.2	3%
Maalox Anti-Diarrheal	8.7	8.3	8.3	•
Parepectolin	7.9	7.6	7.5	1%
Pepto-Bismol Maximum Strength	7.2	7.0	6.8	1%
No Recommendation				2%

• *Indicates that this product was recommended by less than 1% of pharmacists surveyed.*
Bold type indicates the highest rating.

Pharmacists Say...

DIARRHEA CAN LEAD TO DEHYDRATION, especially in the elderly. Therefore, It is important to drink fluids. Try frequent sips of electrolyte drinks such as Gatorade or other sports drinks.

PRODUCTS CONTAINING LOPERAMIDE, such as Imodium A-D and Maalox Anti-Diarrheal, are the most effective for both cramping and diarrhea. However, do not exceed the recommended dosage, because at higher doses it can cause constipation.

DO NOT OVERUSE any of these products or use them for prolonged periods.

PRODUCTS CONTAINING BISMUTH SUBSALICYLATE, such as Pepto-Bismol, contain salicylate and should be avoided by anyone who has been warned not to take aspirin or salicylates.

GENERIC EQUIVALENTS are available for these products. They are less expensive and just as effective as the name brands.

See Your Doctor...

If diarrhea persists for more than 48 hours, or if you experience weakness, dizziness, lightheadedness, lethargy, confusion, bloody stools, fever, nausea, vomiting, or extreme thirst, contact your doctor immediately.

Dry Eyes

Dry eyes occur when the body doesn't produce enough tears to keep the eyes lubricated. The condition can be caused for a number of reasons, including certain medications or prolonged exposure to wind or dry air. If you suffer from dry eyes, be sure to keep air conditioning and heating vents pointed away from you, and use a humidifier to keep air moist. If you wear contact lenses, consult your ophthalmologist before using any of the eyedrops described below.

SYMPTOMS: *Dry, itchy eyes*

| | Rated on a scale of 1 to 10 | | | Percentage Of Pharmacists Who Most Often Recommend |
	Speed Of Relief	Most Effective	Desirable Duration Of Relief	
AquaSite	8.6	8.3	7.5	2%
Celluvisc	8.8	**8.8**	**7.9**	6%
Clear Eyes Lubricant Eye Redness Reliever	8.1	7.7	7.1	•
Dry Eye Therapy	8.3	8.1	7.1	•
HypoTears	**8.9**	8.7	7.7	23%
Liquifilm Tears Lubricant Ophthalmic Solution	8.8	8.5	7.6	3%
Moisture Drops	8.7	8.4	7.3	3%
Murine Tears	8.6	8.2	7.3	8%
Ocurest Tears Formula Lubricant	8.4	8.1	6.9	•
Refresh	8.8	8.6	7.7	11%
Tears Naturale	**8.9**	8.7	7.8	**26%**
No Recommendation				20%

• Indicates that this product was recommended by less than 1% of pharmacists surveyed.
Bold type indicates the highest rating.

Pharmacists Say...

USE OINTMENTS AND VISCOUS DROPS only at night, since they may cloud your vision.

AQUASITE, CELLUVISC, AND REFRESH are packaged in single-use containers and are more expensive than similar products in different packaging.

IF YOU HAVE SENSITIVE EYES, choose products that are free of preservatives.

DON'T USE ANY SOLUTION that's cloudy or has changed color.

See Your Doctor...

If your condition worsens or persists for more than 72 hours, or if you experience eye pain, changes in vision, continued redness, or irritation of the eye, contact your doctor.

See also *Eye Redness*

Dry Skin

Dry skin occurs when the body can't produce enough moisture to keep the outer layers of the skin sufficiently lubricated, and often occurs during the winter when relative humidity is very low. If you have a tendency toward dry skin, use mild soaps to wash your hands and body, and follow up with a good moisturizer. Exposure to hot water can make dry skin worse, so avoid long, hot baths (use lukewarm water instead). Dry skin involving only the hands would benefit from wearing protective gloves to prevent exposure to harsh household detergents.

SYMPTOMS: *Dry, painful areas of skin • Areas of red, scaly, cracking, or peeling skin*

	Rated on a scale of 1 to 10			Percentage Of Pharmacists Who Most Often Recommend
	Most Effective	**Speed Of Relief**	**Desirable Duration Of Relief**	
Aveeno Moisturizing	7.7	8.0	7.4	•
Cetaphil	7.7	7.7	7.3	2%
Curél Therapeutic Moisturizing	8.0	8.0	7.6	5%
Dermasil Dry Skin Treatment	8.1	8.1	7.6	1%
Eucerin Dry Skin Therapy Original	**8.6**	**8.3**	**8.1**	**36%**
Jergens Advanced Therapy Dry Skin Care	7.6	7.6	7.2	1%
Keri Original	8.0	8.0	7.6	3%
Lubriderm Skin Therapy Moisturizing Lotion	8.2	8.1	7.6	14%
Moisturel Skin Protectant Lotion	8.2	8.1	7.7	10%
Neutrogena Emulsion	8.1	8.2	7.8	3%
Nivea Creme Ultra Moisturizing	8.0	8.1	7.8	2%
Pacquin Medicated Hand & Body	7.3	7.7	7.2	•
Vaseline Intensive Care Extra Strength	7.7	7.9	7.3	12%
No Recommendation				12%

• Indicates that this product was recommended by less than 1% of pharmacists surveyed.
Bold type indicates the highest rating.

continued on next page

See also *Dermatitis*

CHOOSE THE PRODUCTS that contain the least number of ingredients, since they'll have fewer chemicals that could irritate your skin.

DIFFERENT PRODUCTS WORK WELL FOR DIFFERENT PEOPLE, so you might have to try a few products before you find the one that works best for you.

IF YOU HAVE SENSITIVE SKIN, try Cetaphil, which is fragrance-free and nongreasy.

THE TREATMENT OF DRY SKIN may require multiple applications of moisturizer daily.

If your dry skin persists or worsens after four weeks of using over-the-counter products, or if a rash develops in addition to the dry skin, contact your doctor.

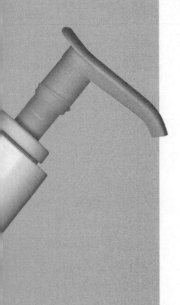

Earwax

Wax is produced in the outer ear canal. If too much of it is produced, the ear canal can become clogged. If you have a buildup of ear wax, don't try to remove it using a cotton swab or other object—you may pack the wax further into the ear, causing damage. Irrigating the ear with warm water or hydrogen peroxide may be all that you need to loosen and remove the wax.

SYMPTOMS: *Feeling that the ear is "plugged" • Impaired hearing or ringing in the affected ear • Itching in the ear • Earache*

	Rated on a scale of 1 to 10			Percentage Of Pharmacists Who Most Often Recommend
	Most Effective	**Ease Of Use**	**Speed Of Relief**	
Auro-Dri Ear Drops	8.1	7.6	7.3	•
Debrox Drops Earwax Removal Aid	**8.7**	**8.1**	**7.7**	**50%**
Murine Earwax Removal System	**8.7**	8.0	**7.7**	47%
No Recommendation				3%

• Indicates that this product was recommended by less than 1% of pharmacists surveyed.
Bold type indicates the highest rating.

Pharmacists Say...

IF YOU HAVE HAD AN EAR INFECTION that caused a perforated ear drum or if you have "tubes" in your ears, contact your doctor before using these products.

ALL THE PRODUCTS IN THIS SECTION are equivalent. The active ingredient is carbamide peroxide, which is also available as a generic medication.

See Your Doctor...

If you experience any loss of hearing, or have ear pain, fever, drainage, or dizziness, contact your doctor.

Eye Redness

Red eyes can be caused by allergies, sleeplessness, and irritation from environmental irritants such as dust. Eye redness is also a symptom of dry eyes; see 'Dry Eyes' on page 66 for more information about treating that ailment. Before using eyedrops, be sure that there are no foreign objects in the eye that are causing the redness. If you wear contact lenses, consult your ophthalmologist before using the eyedrops described below.

SYMPTOMS: *Red, bloodshot eyes • Tearing*

	Rated on a scale of 1 to 10			Percentage Of Pharmacists Who Most Often Recommend
	Most Effective	**Speed Of Relief**	**Minimal Side Effects**	
Clear Eyes Lubricant Eye Redness Reliever	**8.6**	8.5	**8.0**	16%
Murine Tears Plus	**8.6**	8.5	7.8	14%
OcuClear Eye Redness Reliever	8.5	8.5	7.8	9%
Visine Original	**8.6**	**8.6**	**8.0**	**50%**
No Recommendation				11%

Bold type indicates the highest rating.

Pharmacists Say...

BE CAREFUL NOT TO USE these eyedrops for more than a few days at a time. Otherwise you can suffer from "rebound redness."

DO NOT USE THESE PRODUCTS if the solution is outdated or dirty. Do not use them if you wear contact lenses.

THE ABOVE PRODUCTS are for the cosmetic removal of eye redness. If the redness is a result of allergies, try taking an oral antihistamine such as Benadryl and using lubricant eyedrops such as HypoTears or Tears Naturale to soothe your eyes. Lubricant eyedrops can be used as often as necessary since they contain no medication to cause "rebound redness." (If you take an oral antihistamine such as Benadryl, see 'General Warnings' on page xiii regarding antihistamines). If the redness is a result of eye fatigue and overuse, you should use lubricant eyedrops only.

PATIENTS WITH GLAUCOMA or any other chronic eye condition should consult their doctor before using any of these products.

See Your Doctor...

If the condition worsens or persists for more than 72 hours, or if you experience eye pain, changes in vision, continued redness, or irritation of the eye, contact your doctor.

See also *Dry Eyes*

F*ever*

A fever is a common response to a number of different infections and most likely plays a role in the body's attempt to fight off an illness. The majority of fevers resolve themselves within a couple of days. However, there are instances when a fever can be serious or even life threatening. Please refer to "See Your Doctor" at the end of this entry on page 73 for advice on when to contact your doctor immediately.

SYMPTOMS: *Body temperature of more than 100°F (38°C)*

For Adults

	Rated on a scale of 1 to 10			Percentage Of Pharmacists Who Most Often Recommend
	Most Effective	Speed Of Relief	Minimal Side Effects	
Advil	**8.8**	8.2	7.1	13%
Aleve	8.2	7.7	6.7	1%
Anacin Maximum Strength	8.6	8.2	7.2	2%
Ascriptin Maximum Strength	8.4	8.1	7.2	1%
Bayer Aspirin Extra Strength	8.7	**8.3**	7.0	7%
Bufferin Extra Strength	8.5	8.2	7.0	1%
Ecotrin Maximum Strength	8.3	7.4	7.4	1%
Motrin IB	8.7	8.2	7.1	5%
Nuprin Pain Relief Formula	8.7	8.2	7.0	•
Tylenol Extra Strength	**8.8**	**8.3**	**8.8**	**61%**
Orudis KT	8.0	7.5	6.6	•
No Recommendation				9%

• *Indicates that this product was recommended by less than 1% of pharmacists surveyed.*
Bold type indicates the highest rating.

continued on next page

See also *Colds; Flu*

Pharmacists Say...

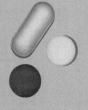

MAKE SURE YOU DRINK PLENTY OF FLUIDS when you have a fever, to prevent dehydration.

COOL BATHS AND SHOWERS can help reduce a fever.

IF YOU HAVE A HISTORY OF PEPTIC ULCERS, bleeding disorders, kidney disease, or asthma, contact your doctor before taking an over-the-counter anti-inflammatory medication such as aspirin, ibuprofen, naproxen, etc.

IF YOU ARE TAKING OTHER MEDICATION, check with your pharmacist or doctor about possible interactions before you take any of these products.

ADVIL, NUPRIN, AND MOTRIN IB are identical products containing 200 mg of ibuprofen.

TAKE ANY ANTI-INFLAMMATORY MEDICATION such as aspirin, ibuprofen, naproxen, etc., with food to avoid upsetting your stomach.

GENERIC EQUIVALENTS are available for these products. They are less expensive and just as effective as the name brands.

For Children

	Rated on a scale of 1 to 10			Percentage Of Pharmacists Who Most Often Recommend
	Most Effective	Desirable Duration Of Relief	Speed Of Relief	
Advil Children's	**9.1**	**8.6**	**8.6**	3%
Motrin Children's	**9.1**	**8.6**	**8.6**	28%
Panadol Children's	8.5	7.9	8.3	•
Tempra 2	8.6	8.0	8.4	1%
Tylenol Children's	8.8	8.1	8.5	**63%**
No Recommendation				6%

• Indicates that this product was recommended by less than 1% of pharmacists surveyed.

Bold type indicates the highest rating.

BECAUSE ACETAMINOPHEN has fewer side effects, it is the treatment of choice for children with fever.

BECAUSE OF THE RISK of Reye's Syndrome, don't give children any product that contains aspirin.

DO NOT USE ALCOHOL BATHS to cool a child who has a fever; instead, try bathing the child in lukewarm water.

IF YOUR CHILD HAS A HISTORY of bleeding disorders, kidney disease, or asthma, contact a doctor before giving your child any product containing ibuprofen. (Refer to Section Two, 'About The Products,' on page 131, for information on the active ingredients for the above products.)

GENERIC EQUIVALENTS are available for these products. They are less expensive and just as effective as the name brands.

If you have a temperature of 101° that persists for more than 3 days, or if you have a fever of 103° or greater, contact your doctor. If your fever is associated with a severe headache, stiff neck, confusion, severe swelling of the throat, shortness of breath, abdominal pain, painful urination, or joint pain, contact your doctor immediately. Furthermore, a low-grade fever without any other symptoms that persists for more than two weeks warrants a medical evaluation.

WARNING: The elderly and children are very susceptible to dehydration when they develop fevers; therefore, any symptoms of dehydration require immediate attention. Symptoms of dehydration include dizziness, weakness, lethargy, confusion, irritability, or any change in mental status, increased thirst, dark yellow urine, or diminished amounts of urine.

Flatulence

Flatulence occurs from the production of gas by bacteria as they break down food and its by-products. Foods such as beans, broccoli, and cabbage can result in excessive production of gas. Flatulence can also be a symptom of a mild lactose intolerance. If you regularly suffer from this ailment, consider carefully monitoring the foods that you eat to identify the likely causes.

SYMPTOMS: *Frequent passing of gas*

| | Rated on a scale of 1 to 10 | | | Percentage Of Pharmacists Who Most Often Recommend |
	Most Effective	Speed Of Relief	Minimal Side Effects	
Beano	7.4	6.8	8.4	8%
CharcoCaps	6.6	6.2	7.3	1%
Gas-X	8.3	7.9	8.9	22%
Maalox Anti-Gas Regular Strength	8.0	7.7	8.8	1%
Mylanta Gas Relief	**8.4**	**8.0**	**9.0**	**46%**
Phazyme Gas Relief (95mg)	**8.4**	7.9	8.9	17%
No Recommendation				6%

Bold type indicates the highest rating.

Pharmacists Say...

BEANO is more of a preventive product than the others and is particularly effective in reducing flatulence associated with high-fiber diets.

GENERIC EQUIVALENTS are available for these products. They are less expensive and just as effective as the name brands.

See Your Doctor...

If you've tried using over-the-counter medications and have not obtained relief, contact your doctor.

F*lu*

The flu is an infectious disease caused by a virus that's easily spread by coughs, sneezes, or hand-to-hand contact. There are many different strains of the flu virus; although vaccinations are available to help prevent you from catching some of the most common types, these vaccinations are good only against specific strains of flu and are effective for only one season. If you have the flu, rest and drink plenty of liquids to ensure that you don't become dehydrated.

SYMPTOMS: *Body aches • Fever • Congestion • Coughing • Sore throat*

For Adults

With body aches **and** *fever:*

PAIN RELIEVERS

	Rated on a scale of 1 to 10			Percentage Of Pharmacists Who Most Often Recommend
	Most Effective	Speed Of Relief	Minimal Side Effects	
Advil	**8.8**	**8.2**	7.1	30%
Aleve	8.4	7.7	6.7	3%
Anacin Maximum Strength	8.3	8.1	7.0	2%
Ascriptin Maximum Strength	8.2	7.9	7.2	2%
Bayer Aspirin Extra Strength	8.4	8.0	6.9	3%
Bufferin Extra Strength	8.3	7.9	7.1	2%
Ecotrin Maximum Strength	8.2	7.2	7.3	1%
Motrin IB	**8.8**	**8.2**	7.1	7%
Nuprin Pain Relief Formula	**8.8**	**8.2**	7.0	•
Orudis KT	8.3	7.8	6.6	1%
Tylenol Extra Strength	8.2	8.0	**8.8**	**44%**
No Recommendation				6%

• *Indicates that this product was recommended by less than 1% of pharmacists surveyed.*
Bold type indicates the highest rating.

continued on next page

See also *Colds; Coughs; Fever; Sore Throat*

COOL BATHS AND SHOWERS can help reduce a fever.

IF YOU HAVE A HISTORY OF PEPTIC ULCERS, bleeding disorders, kidney disease, or asthma, contact your doctor before taking an over-the-counter anti-inflammatory medication such as aspirin, ibuprofen, naproxen, etc.

IF YOU ARE TAKING OTHER MEDICATION, check with your pharmacist or doctor about possible interactions before you take any of these products.

ADVIL, NUPRIN, AND MOTRIN IB are identical products containing 200 mg of ibuprofen.

TAKE ANY ANTI-INFLAMMATORY MEDICATION such as aspirin, ibuprofen, naproxen, etc., with food to avoid upsetting your stomach.

GENERIC EQUIVALENTS are available for these products. They are less expensive and just as effective as the name brands.

With body aches, fever, **and** *congestion:*

ANTIHISTIMINE, DECONGESTANT, PAIN RELIEVER COMBINATIONS

	Rated on a scale of 1 to 10			Percentage Of Pharmacists Who Most Often Recommend
	Most Effective	Speed Of Relief	Minimal Side Effects	
Actifed Cold & Sinus	**8.6**	8.1	7.3	**35%**
Benadryl Allergy/Cold	8.0	7.8	6.9	4%
Coricidin 'D'	7.8	7.7	7.3	4%
Dimetapp Allergy Sinus	8.1	7.8	**7.4**	10%
Drixoral Cold & Flu 12 Hour Relief	8.3	7.8	**7.4**	10%
TheraFlu Flu And Cold Medicine Original Formula	8.3	**8.4**	**7.4**	20%
No Recommendation				17%

Bold type indicates the highest rating.

With body aches, fever, congestion, **and** *cough:*

ANTIHISTAMINE, DECONGESTANT/PAIN RELIEVER, COUGH SUPPRESSANT COMBINATIONS

	Rated on a scale of 1 to 10			Percentage Of Pharmacists Who Most Often Recommend
	Most Effective	**Speed Of Relief**	**Minimal Side Effects**	
Comtrex Maximum Strength Multi-Symptom Cold & Flu Relief	8.3	7.8	7.1	20%
Contac Severe Cold & Flu Maximum Strength	8.0	7.6	6.8	1%
Robitussin Night-Time Cold Formula	8.2	7.8	**7.5**	17%
TheraFlu Maximum Strength Flu, Cold & Cough Medicine NightTime	**8.4**	**8.2**	7.2	12%
Tylenol Cold Multi-Symptom	**8.4**	7.9	**7.5**	**21%**
Vicks 44M Cough, Cold & Flu Relief	8.0	7.8	6.9	2%
Vicks Nyquil Multi-Symptom Cold/Flu Relief	8.2	8.1	6.7	11%
No Recommendation				15%

Bold type indicates the highest rating.

Pharmacists Say...

COMBINATION PRODUCTS CONTAIN MANY INGREDIENTS. If you take such a product you may be taking more medication than you need and subjecting yourself to unnecessary side effects. Treat only the symptoms that you actually have.

COMBINATION PRODUCTS containing an antihistamine can cause drowsiness and are best used at night, since they can help you get adequate rest.

PRODUCTS THAT YOU MIX WITH HOT WATER to form a warm drink have no advantage over pills with similar ingredients and are much more expensive. Sipping a hot drink at the same time you take a pill provides the same effect for less money.

IF YOU HAVE A BREATHING PROBLEM such as emphysema or chronic bronchitis or have heart disease, high blood pressure, thyroid disease, diabetes, glaucoma, or prostate disease, contact your pharmacist or doctor before taking any product containing both an antihistamine and a decongestant.

DO NOT CRUSH OR CHEW A LONG-ACTING PRODUCT. Swallow whole to prevent a sudden release of excessive medication.

continued on next page

IF YOU ARE TAKING OTHER MEDICATION, check with your pharmacist or doctor about possible interactions before you take these products.

GENERIC EQUIVALENTS are available for these products. They are less expensive and just as effective as the name brands.

For Children

*With body aches **and** fever:*

PAIN RELIEVERS

| | Rated on a scale of 1 to 10 | | | Percentage Of Pharmacists Who Most Often Recommend |
	Most Effective	Desirable Duration Of Relief	Speed Of Relief	
Advil Children's	**9.0**	**8.5**	8.3	5%
Motrin Children's	**9.0**	**8.5**	8.3	29%
Panadol Children's	8.3	7.8	8.2	•
Tempra 2	8.4	7.8	8.2	1%
Tylenol Children's	8.6	8.0	**8.4**	**59%**
No Recommendation				7%

• *Indicates that this product was recommended by less than 1% of pharmacists surveyed.*
Bold type indicates the highest rating.

Pharmacists Say...

BECAUSE ACETAMINOPHEN has fewer side effects, it is the treatment of choice for children with fever.

BECAUSE OF THE RISK of Reye's Syndrome, don't give children any product that contains aspirin.

DO NOT USE ALCOHOL BATHS to cool a child who has a fever; instead, try bathing the child in lukewarm water.

IF YOUR CHILD HAS A HISTORY of bleeding disorders, kidney disease, or asthma, contact a doctor before giving your child any product containing ibuprofen. (Refer to Section Two, 'About The Products,' on page 131, for information on the active ingredients for the above products.)

GENERIC EQUIVALENTS are available for these products. They are less expensive and just as effective as the name brands.

With body aches, fever, **and** *congestion:*

ANTIHISTAMINE, DECONGESTANT, PAIN RELIEVER COMBINATIONS

| | Rated on a scale of 1 to 10 | | | Percentage Of Pharmacists Who Most Often Recommend |
	Most Effective	Desirable Duration Of Relief	Speed Of Relief	
Tylenol Children's Cold Multi Symptom	**8.4**	**7.8**	**8.0**	**65%**
No Recommendation				35%

With bodyaches, fever, congestion, **and** *cough:*

ANTIHISTAMINE, DECONGESTANT, PAIN RELIEVER, COUGH SUPPRESSANT COMBINATIONS

| | Rated on a scale of 1 to 10 | | | Percentage Of Pharmacists Who Most Often Recommend |
	Most Effective	Desirable Duration Of Relief	Speed Of Relief	
Triaminic* Sore Throat Pain & Cough	8.1	**7.7**	7.9	18%
Tylenol Children's Cold Multi Symptom Plus Cough	**8.4**	**7.7**	**8.0**	**56%**
No Recommendation				26%

*This product does not contain an antihistamine, and so does not cause drowsiness.

Bold type indicates the highest rating.

Pharmacists Say...

COMBINATION PRODUCTS CONTAIN MANY INGREDIENTS. If you give your children such a product you may be giving them more medication than they need and subjecting them to unnecessary side effects. Treat only the symptoms that they actually have.

PRODUCTS THAT CONTAIN AN ANTIHISTAMINE usually cause drowsiness. However, antihistamines may cause some children to become hyperactive.

IF YOUR CHILD HAS A HISTORY OF ASTHMA, chronic lung disease, heart disease, high blood pressure, diabetes, thyroid disease, or difficulty in urination, contact a doctor before giving your child any product containing both an antihistamine and a decongestant.

GENERIC EQUIVALENTS are available for these products. They are less expensive and just as effective as the name brands.

See Your Doctor...

The flu can be a serious condition. You should see your doctor if your symptoms worsen or do not improve within seven days, or recur after initial improvement. Patients with chronic medical conditions may want to contact their doctor immediately if they develop symptoms of the flu.

Hangover

Drinking alcohol can cause a variety of ailments to occur "the morning after." Headache, nausea, indigestion, exhaustion, and muscle pain are some of the symptoms that develop after excessive consumption of alcohol. While you're drinking, you can decrease your chance of a hangover by not drinking on an empty stomach, and by sticking to clear liquors such as vodka, which have fewer hangover-causing impurities. After you're finished drinking alcohol, be sure to drink plenty of water before you go to bed and first thing in the morning to avoid dehydration. If your preventive measures don't work and you wake up with a hangover, drink fruit juice or eat some jam or honey, which may alleviate some of your symptoms.

SYMPTOMS: *Headache • Nausea • Indigestion • Exhaustion*

	Rated on a scale of 1 to 10			Percentage Of Pharmacists Who Most Often Recommend
	Most Effective	**Speed Of Relief**	**Minimal Side Effects**	
Advil	**7.4**	7.2	6.7	16%
Aleve	7.0	6.9	6.3	5%
Alka Seltzer Original	**7.4**	**7.9**	7.4	26%
Ascriptin Maximum Strength	7.2	7.0	6.9	1%
Bayer Aspirin Extra Strength	7.3	7.2	6.8	2%
Bufferin Extra Strength	7.3	7.2	6.9	3%
Ecotrin Maximum Strength	7.0	6.5	6.9	1%
Maalox Extra Strength Antacid/Anti-Gas	6.0	6.8	**7.8**	1%
Motrin IB	**7.4**	7.2	6.7	1%
Mylanta Maximum Strength Fast Acting Antacid/Anti-Gas	6.0	6.8	**7.8**	2%
Nuprin Pain Relief Formula	**7.4**	7.2	6.7	•
Orudis KT	7.0	6.9	6.3	1%
Tylenol Extra Strength	7.3	7.2	**7.8**	**30%**
No Recommendation				12%

• Indicates that this product was recommended by less than 1% of pharmacists surveyed.
Bold type indicates the highest rating.

ANTI-INFLAMMATORY MEDICATIONS such as aspirin, ibuprofen, or naproxen, etc., may irritate an already inflamed stomach. These products should not be taken by anyone with a history of peptic ulcers, bleeding disorders, kidney disease, or asthma, without first consulting a doctor.

TRY TREATING THE SYMPTOMS of a hangover individually—if you have a headache, take an analgesic; if you have heartburn, take an antacid. (Refer to Section Two, 'About The Products,' on page 131, for information on the active ingredients for the above products. Then see Section Three, the 'Glossary,' on page 175, for an explanation of those ingredients.)

GENERIC EQUIVALENTS are available for these products. They are less expensive and just as effective as the name brands.

A hangover rarely requires medical attention.

Headache

Headaches are one of the most common ailments and have multiple causes. The most common headache is the tension headache, which occurs as a result of stress and fatigue. Headaches can also be caused by a variety of illnesses, such as sinus infection, TMJ (temporomandibular joint) disorder, and hangovers. Migraines are a special category of headache discussed in more detail on page 98. Nonmedicinal measures that can help headaches include neck and temple massages, cool compresses on the forehead, or warm compresses on the back of the neck. If your headache is due to allergies, see the chart and tips on page 7. If your headache is due to colds, see the chart and tips on page 31.

SYMPTOMS: *Pain, ranging from a dull generalized ache to a sharp localized pain*

| | Rated on a scale of 1 to 10 | | | Percentage Of Pharmacists Who Most Often Recommend |
	Most Effective	Speed Of Relief	Minimal Side Effects	
Advil	**8.7**	**8.2**	7.1	28%
Aleve	8.5	7.9	6.8	6%
Anacin Maximum Strength	8.5	**8.2**	7.1	3%
Ascriptin Maximum Strength	8.3	8.0	7.3	•
Bayer Aspirin Extra Strength	8.4	**8.2**	7.0	8%
Bufferin Extra Strength	8.4	8.1	7.3	2%
Ecotrin Maximum Strength	8.0	7.2	7.5	1%
Motrin IB	**8.7**	8.1	7.1	7%
Nuprin Pain Relief Formula	**8.7**	8.1	7.1	•
Tylenol Extra Strength	8.3	8.1	**8.7**	35%
Orudis KT	8.4	7.8	6.7	1%
No Recommendation				10%

• *Indicates that this product was recommended by less than 1% of pharmacists surveyed.*
Bold type indicates the highest rating.

See also *Migraine*

ADVIL, NUPRIN, AND MOTRIN IB are identical products containing 200 mg of ibuprofen.

IF YOU ARE TAKING OTHER MEDICATION, check with your pharmacist or doctor about possible interactions before you take any of these products.

IF YOU HAVE A HISTORY OF PEPTIC ULCERS, bleeding disorders, kidney disease, or asthma, contact your doctor before taking an over-the-counter anti-inflammatory medication such as aspirin, ibuprofen, naproxen, etc.

TAKE ANY ANTI-INFLAMMATORY MEDICATION such as aspirin, ibuprofen, naproxen, etc., with food to avoid upsetting your stomach.

GENERIC EQUIVALENTS are available for these products. They are less expensive and just as effective as the name brands.

Any headache that is severe, persists for more than two days, recurs frequently or is associated with neurologic symptoms such as numbness, weakness, loss of vision, or clumsiness should be seen by a doctor immediately.

Head Lice

Head lice are small insects that live in hair; the itching associated with lice is a result of their bites. Lice are often spread among schoolchildren and are considered a public health hazard; if your child has lice, you should inform the school immediately. In addition to the treatments below, be sure to wash hairbrushes, combs, hats, and other items that came into contact with the infected person, in very hot water, and dry them in a hot dryer. If it's not possible to wash these items, they should definitely be thrown out.

SYMPTOMS: *Visible insects in the hair • Visible insect eggs, called "nits" • Itching of the scalp and affected areas*

	Rated on a scale of 1 to 10			Percentage Of Pharmacists Who Most Often Recommend
	Most Effective	**Speed Of Relief**	**Ease Of Use**	
A-200 Lice Killing Shampoo	8.4	8.2	8.0	6%
Clear Total Lice Treatment Elimination System	7.6	7.9	7.8	•
Nix Lice Treatment	**9.3**	**8.8**	**8.7**	**82%**
Pronto Lice Killing Shampoo	8.2	8.0	7.8	•
Rid Maximum Strength Lice-Killing Shampoo	8.5	8.3	8.1	10%
Tegrin-LT Lice Treatment Shampoo/Conditioner	7.8	7.9	7.3	•
Tisit	8.0	7.9	7.7	•
No Recommendation				3%

• Indicates that this product was recommended by less than 1% of pharmacists surveyed.
Bold type indicates the highest rating.

NIX SEEMS TO HAVE some preventive effects as well as being an effective treatment.

USE A COMB TO REMOVE THE NITS from the affected person's head. Check all the members of your family for head lice and treat everyone who's affected.

ALL OF THESE PRODUCTS must be used on dry or nearly dry hair. Wet hair will dilute the medication, and it won't work as effectively as it should.

If there is no improvement from over-the-counter medications or if skin irritation occurs as a result of these products, contact your doctor.

Heartburn

The sensation of heartburn is caused by acid reflux, which occurs when stomach acid leaks upward into the esophagus (the passage that food travels between your mouth and your stomach). Acid reflux can be caused by eating too much food, by eating too quickly, or by eating foods that are fatty, greasy, or fried. Caffeine, chocolate, citrus juice, and spicy foods can also trigger heartburn for some people. A simple remedy that may relieve some heartburn is to loosen your clothes—a tight belt or waistline can squeeze your stomach, causing acid to flow up to the esophagus. To prevent heartburn while sleeping, don't eat for two hours before bedtime, and try raising the head of your bed with two to four inch blocks.

SYMPTOMS: *Painful burning sensation beneath the rib cage after eating or during the night • Acid taste with belching*

	Rated on a scale of 1 to 10			Percentage Of Pharmacists Who Most Often Recommend
	Most Effective	**Speed Of Relief**	**Minimal Side Effects**	
Di-Gel Antacid/Anti-Gas Liquid	7.7	8.1	8.2	•
Gaviscon Extra Strength Liquid Antacid	8.3	8.5	8.4	13%
Maalox Heartburn Relief	8.3	8.6	8.3	4%
Mylanta Maximum Strength Fast Acting Antacid/Anti-Gas	8.4	**8.7**	8.3	25%
Pepcid AC Acid Controller	**9.1**	7.7	**8.5**	**36%**
Riopan Plus Double Strength Antacid & Anti-Gas Liquid	8.1	8.4	8.3	1%
Rolaids Antacid Tablets	7.5	7.8	8.2	•
Tagamet HB 200	8.8	7.5	7.3	1%
Tums E-X Extra Strength	7.7	7.9	8.3	6%
Zantac 75	9.0	7.7	8.4	9%
No Recommendation				6%

• *Indicates that this product was recommended by less than 1% of pharmacists surveyed.*
Bold type indicates the highest rating.

Also see *Indigestion*

PEPCID AC, TAGAMET HB 200, AND ZANTAC 75 are best used for preventing indigestion and heartburn instead of treating it. These products may not take effect for 30 to 60 minutes after you take them. If you already have the symptoms of heartburn, an antacid will provide the fastest relief, but the effects won't be as strong or as long lasting as if you had used a preventive medication.

LIQUID ANTACIDS tend to provide relief from indigestion and heartburn more quickly than tablets.

PATIENTS WITH KIDNEY DISEASE should check with their doctor or pharmacist before taking any antacids.

GENERIC EQUIVALENTS are available for some of these products. They are less expensive and just as effective as the name brands.

If your heartburn persists for more than one week despite taking the recommended maximum dosage of over-the-counter medications, or if you have abdominal pain, contact your doctor.

WARNING: Angina or heart attack can sometimes be confused with heartburn! If you have any of the symptoms of a heart problem in addition to the heartburn (such as dizziness, shortness of breath, clammy skin, or nausea), you should get immediate medical attention.

Hemorrhoids

Hemorrhoids are swollen veins around the anus, which are most frequently caused by straining while attempting to pass a stool. If you suffer from hemorrhoids, try to avoid constipation by eating a high-fiber diet, drinking plenty of liquids, and exercising regularly. In addition to the medications listed below, be sure to clean yourself gently and carefully after a bowel movement to keep the tissues from becoming more irritated. Many people report relief after sitting for ten or fifteen minutes in a "sitz bath"—a tub half-filled with warm (not hot) water.

SYMPTOMS: *Bowel movements that are painful as they pass through the anus • Rectal itching • Rectal bleeding (visible on the toilet paper)*

| | Rated on a scale of 1 to 10 | | | Percentage Of Pharmacists Who Most Often Recommend |
	Most Effective	Speed Of Relief	Ease Of Use	
Americaine Hemorrhoidal Ointment	8.0	**8.6**	8.1	6%
Anusol Hemorrhoidal Ointment	8.0	7.8	8.0	**30%**
Cortizone-10	8.0	7.6	7.9	16%
Hemorid For Women Hemorrhoidal Creme	7.5	7.6	7.9	2%
Preparation H	7.5	7.4	8.0	19%
Tronolane	**8.1**	8.3	7.9	10%
Tucks Medicated Pads	7.2	7.8	**8.6**	5%
No Recommendation				12%

Bold type indicates the highest rating.

FOR BEST RELIEF, dissolve Epsom salts in bath water that's as hot as you can sit in comfortably. After soaking for 15 to 20 minutes, apply the medication of your choice.

CHOOSE YOUR MEDICATION based on the symptoms you're experiencing. If your primary complaint is pain or burning, an anesthetic may be best. If your primary complaint is inflammation or itching, a hydrocortisone product may be better. (Refer to Section Two, 'About The Products,' on page 131, for information on the active ingredients for the above products. Then refer to Section Three, the 'Glossary,' on page 175, for an explanation of those ingredients.)

Hemorrhoids should be diagnosed by your doctor. If you have severe pain or excessive bleeding, or if your symptoms recur frequently, or do not improve, contact your doctor. Blood in the stools, especially in people over the age of 50, may indicate a more serious condition than hemorrhoids.

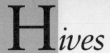# Hives

Hives are raised, red, often itchy welts that are caused by the release of histamines. This immune response can be triggered by a variety of factors, including food, food additives, medications, and physical factors such as exposure to cold or sunlight. Hives may also be triggered by a number of infections. In addition to the medications listed below, a cool compress will relieve itching and reduce swelling.

SYMPTOMS: *Large, raised, red itchy lumps on the skin that rise, then subside in a few hours*

	Rated on a scale of 1 to 10			Percentage Of Pharmacists Who Most Often Recommend
	Speed Of Relief	Most Effective	Desirable Duration Of Relief	
Benadryl Allergy	**8.7**	**9.2**	7.9	**89%**
Chlor-Trimeton Allergy 8 Hour	7.3	7.7	7.8	1%
Chlor-Trimeton Allergy 12 Hour	7.3	7.8	**8.2**	1%
Dimetapp Allergy	7.6	7.5	7.4	•
Efidac/24 Chlorpheniramine	6.9	7.3	8.0	•
Tavist-1	7.5	7.8	8.0	7%
No Recommendation				3%

• *Indicates that this product was recommended by less than 1% of pharmacists surveyed.*
Bold type indicates the highest rating.

Pharmacists Say...

ALL THE PRODUCTS listed in this section are antihistamines and have similar effects. If antihistamines make you drowsy, try a product that contains chlorpheniramine—this chemical is less sedating than other antihistamines. (Refer to Section Two, 'About The Products,' on page 131, for information on the active ingredients for the above products.)

DIPHENHYDRAMINE, the active ingredient in Benadryl, is the best medication for treating hives; however, it will almost certainly make you drowsy.

IF YOU HAVE GLAUCOMA, prostate disease, or breathing problems such as emphysema or chronic bronchitis, contact your pharmacist or doctor before taking any product containing an antihistamine.

YOU CAN RELIEVE the itching associated with hives by applying a topical hydrocortisone product to the affected area.

IN SOME PEOPLE, antihistamines can cause excitability, sleeplessness, or irritability. These side effects may be more common with the elderly.

GENERIC EQUIVALENTS are available for these products. They are less expensive and just as effective as the name brands.

See Your Doctor...

If you experience difficulty breathing, dizziness, or lightheadedness you should contact your doctor immediately. Furthermore, if the hives last for more than 48 hours, or if they recur frequently despite the use of medication, see your doctor.

Indigestion

Indigestion is a general term for abdominal discomfort associated with bloating, belching, and heartburn. It commonly occurs after meals or excessive consumption of alcohol.

SYMPTOMS: *Heartburn • Mild nausea • Belching • Bloating*

| | Rated on a scale of 1 to 10 | | | Percentage Of Pharmacists Who Most Often Recommend |
	Most Effective	Speed Of Relief	Minimal Side Effects	
Alka-Seltzer Original	7.4	8.2	7.3	3%
Di-Gel Antacid/Anti-Gas Liquid	7.7	8.1	8.0	5%
Gaviscon Extra Strength Liquid Antacid	8.1	8.4	**8.4**	16%
Maalox Heartburn Relief	8.4	**8.5**	8.2	15%
Pepcid AC Acid Controller	**8.6**	7.5	**8.4**	**27%**
Pepto-Bismol Maximum Strength	7.5	7.6	7.3	10%
Rolaids Antacid Tablets	7.6	7.6	8.0	3%
Tagamet HB 200	8.4	7.4	7.4	•
Tums E-X Exra Strength	7.7	7.6	8.1	6%
Zantac 75	**8.6**	7.5	8.3	9%
No Recommendation				8%

• Indicates that this product was recommended by less than 1% of pharmacists surveyed.

Bold type indicates the highest rating.

See also *Heartburn*

Pharmacists Say...

LIQUID ANTACIDS tend to provide relief from indigestion and heartburn more quickly than tablets.

PEPCID AC, TAGAMET HB 200, AND ZANTAC 75 are best used for preventing indigestion and heartburn instead of treating it. These products may not take effect for 30 to 60 minutes after you take them. If you already have the symptoms of heartburn, an antacid will provide the fastest relief, but the effects won't be as strong or as long lasting as if you had used a preventive medication.

PATIENTS WITH KIDNEY DISEASE should check with their doctor or pharmacist before taking any antacids.

GENERIC EQUIVALENTS are available for some of these products. They are less expensive and just as effective as the name brands.

See Your Doctor...

If your indigestion lasts for more than two or three days or recurs frequently, contact your doctor. Any indigestion associated with abdominal pain should be seen by a doctor immediately.

WARNING: Angina or a heart attack can sometimes be confused with indigestion! If you have any of the symptoms of a heart problem in addition to the indigestion (such as dizziness, shortness of breath, clammy skin, or nausea), you should get immediate medical attention.

Insect Bites

Although they're irritating, mosquito, ant, and flea bites are usually only a potential health threat if you're allergic to them. Exceptions include Lyme disease, carried by ticks; encephalitis, carried by mosquitoes; and malaria, transmitted by mosquitoes in tropical countries. Preventing insect bites is preferable to treating them after the fact. If you're in a bug-infested area, wear long sleeves and pants, don't wear heavy perfumes, and apply an insect repellent containing DEET to all exposed areas of your body. In addition to the medications listed below, you can stop the itch of an insect bite by applying an ice cube or an unseasoned meat tenderizer.

SYMPTOMS: *Swollen, itchy welts*

| | Rated on a scale of 1 to 10 | | | Percentage Of |
	Most Effective	Speed Of Relief	Desirable Duration Of Relief	Pharmacists Who Most Often Recommend
Aveeno Anti-itch Cream	7.9	**7.9**	7.5	10%
Benadryl Itch Stopping Extra Strength	7.3	7.5	7.1	10%
Caladryl	6.9	7.2	6.8	2%
Cortaid Maximum Strength	**8.4**	**7.9**	**7.8**	**45%**
Dermarest	7.8	7.8	7.4	3%
No Recommendation				31%

Bold type indicates the highest rating.

Pharmacists Say...

FOR THE BEST RELIEF OF SYMPTOMS, try using a hydrocortisone cream or ointment such as Cortaid Maximum Strength on the affected area during the day, and taking an oral antihistamine such as Benadryl or its generic equivalent at night. See 'General Warnings' (page xiii) regarding antihistamines.

PRODUCTS THAT CONTAIN HYDROCORTISONE are more effective and provide longer-lasting relief than products that contain only an anesthetic. (Refer to Section Two, 'About The Products,' on page 131, for information on the active ingredients for the above products.)

GENERIC HYDROCORTISONE is less expensive and equally effective as the name-brand products.

See Your Doctor...

If you have a severe allergic reaction such as swelling, hives, or difficulty breathing, contact your doctor immediately. The development of a rash, fever, or headache several days after an insect bite warrants a medical evaluation.

Insomnia

Nearly everyone suffers an occasional bout of sleeplessness, which can be caused by stress or environmental changes, or simply occur unexpectedly. Some tips for dealing with insomnia include setting a regular sleep schedule seven days a week; taking a warm bath an hour before bedtime; and eating a light snack just before bed. In general, you should avoid alcohol when you can't sleep—although it may help you drop off initially, it can cause you to wake up later and have even more trouble getting to sleep. You should also avoid caffeinated beverages such as coffee, tea, and many kinds of soft drinks for several hours before going to bed.

SYMPTOMS: *Inability to fall asleep*

	Rated on a scale of 1 to 10			Percentage Of Pharmacists Who Most Often Recommend
	Most Effective	**Speed Of Relief**	**Desirable Duration Of Relief**	
Benadryl Allergy	**8.5**	**8.0**	**7.8**	**65%**
Compōz NightTime Sleep Aid Maximum Strength	8.0	7.5	7.4	•
Nervine Nightime Sleep-Aid	7.8	7.5	7.1	•
Nytol Quick Caps	8.2	7.8	7.5	2%
Nytol Maximum Strength Nightime Sleep-Aid	8.3	7.8	7.7	4%
Sleep-eze 3	8.0	7.6	7.3	•
Sleepinal Maximum Strength Night-Time Sleep-Aid	8.3	7.8	7.5	1%
Sominex Maximum Strength	8.3	7.8	7.6	7%
Unisom Nightime Sleep Aid	8.3	7.9	**7.8**	15%
Unisom SleepGels Maximum Strength	8.2	7.8	7.6	2%
No Recommendation				5%

• *Indicates that this product was recommended by less than 1% of pharmacists surveyed.*
Bold type indicates the highest rating.

continued on next page

WHEN YOU'RE CHOOSING A PRODUCT, be sure to compare active ingredients. Over-the-counter medications for insomnia contain either diphenhydramine or doxylamine. (Refer to Section Two, 'About The Products,' on page 131, for information on the active ingredients for the above products.) A generic brand of diphenhydramine will be much less expensive and just as effective as a name-brand product.

DON'T TAKE ANY MORE MEDICATION than the amount recommended on the label. Larger doses won't help you sleep better, but will increase unpleasant side effects like dry mouth, constipation, and urinary problems. These side effects are uncomfortable for anyone but can become significant problems for elderly people.

THESE PRODUCTS SHOULD be used for only a short period of time.

IF YOU HAVE GLAUCOMA, prostate disease, or breathing problems such as emphysema or chronic bronchitis, contact your pharmacist or doctor before taking any product containing an antihistamine.

If your insomnia lasts for more than two weeks, contact your doctor. Persistent insomnia may be a symptom of a serious medical condition.

Jock Itch

Jock itch is caused by a fungal infection that lives in warm, moist areas like the groin. To avoid jock itch, change out of your workout clothes as quickly as possible; wash with antibacterial soap after each workout; and apply talcum powder to the area.

SYMPTOMS: *Red, painful, itchy, or scaly skin in and around the groin and genitals*

	Rated on a scale of 1 to 10			Percentage Of Pharmacists Who Most Often Recommend
	Most Effective	Speed Of Relief	Desirable Duration Of Relief	
Cruex Antifungal	7.8	7.3	7.5	5%
Lotrimin Antifungal AF	**9.1**	**8.0**	**8.2**	**64%**
Micatin	8.7	7.8	8.1	11%
Tinactin Antifungal	8.4	7.7	7.9	17%
No Recommendation				3%

Bold type indicates the highest rating.

Pharmacists Say...

THE SAME INGREDIENTS that are used to treat jock itch are also used to treat vaginal yeast infections. Lotrimin AF has the same active ingredient as Gyne-Lotrimin and Femstat, while Micatin has the same active ingredient as Monistat. You can compare the costs of the different versions to see which makes the most sense to purchase; however, if you use a vaginal cream to treat jock itch, be sure to write down the instructions for treating jock itch from a package of the product designed for that purpose.

TO ENSURE THAT YOUR CONDITION IS COMPLETELY CURED, keep the affected area as dry as possible, and use the medication for at least one full week after your symptoms are gone.

AFTER YOUR CONDITION CLEARS UP, dust the area daily with talcum powder to absorb excess moisture and decrease the chance of a recurrence.

GENERIC EQUIVALENTS are available for these products. They are less expensive and just as effective as the name brands.

See Your Doctor...

If there is no improvement in your condition within two weeks or if irritation occurs, contact your doctor.

Migraine

No one knows what causes migraines, but they're more likely to occur in women than in men. Migraines may be triggered in some people by certain foods, such as chocolate, nuts, and red wine. Migraine sufferers may find relief by resting in a dark, quiet room and applying a cool compress to the head.

SYMPTOMS: *Sharp pain on one side of the head • Nausea or vomiting • Dizziness • Impaired vision • Extreme sensitivity to sound or light*

	Rated on a scale of 1 to 10			Percentage Of Pharmacists Who Most Often Recommend
	Most Effective	**Speed Of Relief**	**Minimal Side Effects**	
Advil	**7.4**	**7.0**	6.9	**28%**
Aleve	7.3	6.8	6.6	13%
Anacin Maximum Strength	7.0	**7.0**	6.8	6%
Ascriptin Maximum Strength	6.7	6.9	7.0	•
Bayer Aspirin Extra Strength	6.9	6.9	6.8	2%
Bufferin Extra Strength	6.9	6.8	6.9	2%
Ecotrin Maximum Strength	6.5	6.2	7.1	2%
Motrin IB	7.3	**7.0**	6.8	8%
Nuprin Pain Relief Formula	7.3	**7.0**	6.8	2%
Tylenol	6.5	6.7	**8.1**	17%
Orudis KT	7.2	6.9	6.7	3%
No Recommendation				18%

• Indicates that this product was recommended by less than 1% of pharmacists surveyed.
Bold type indicates the highest rating.

See also *Headache*

OVER-THE-COUNTER MEDICATION MAY NOT BE EFFECTIVE FOR THE TREATMENT OF MIGRAINES. If you attempt to use these products, see 'General Warnings' (page xiii) regarding anti-inflammatory medications.

Migraine headaches should always be diagnosed and managed by a doctor. If you have any of the symptoms of a migraine, contact your doctor immediately for advice.

Motion Sickness

Motion sickness is characterized by nausea and vomiting that occurs while riding in any moving vehicle. A discrepancy between what your eyes see and what your inner ear senses can result in conflicting signals to the brain, which leads to nausea. To avoid motion sickness, try to eat small meals before you travel, as traveling on an empty stomach may make you feel worse. If you're susceptible to motion sickness, avoid reading while you travel. Some people report that taking ginger tablets helps them avoid becoming nauseous, while others find some relief in an "acupressure" technique of pressing the thumb against the middle of the wrist or by wearing a wristband that exerts pressure in the same spot.

S Y M P T O M S : *Nausea • Dizziness • Clammy skin • Vomiting*

	Rated on a scale of 1 to 10			Percentage Of Pharmacists Who Most Often Recommend
	Speed Of Relief	**Most Effective**	**Desirable Duration Of Relief**	
Bonine	**8.3**	**8.6**	**8.4**	**48%**
Calm-X	7.5	7.2	6.8	•
Cola Syrup	7.2	6.2	6.0	1%
Dramamine Original Formula	8.2	8.4	7.9	32%
Dramamine II Less Drowsy formula	8.2	8.5	8.3	13%
Emetrol	7.3	6.5	6.3	3%
Nauzene	7.4	7.2	6.9	•
Triptone	7.5	7.4	6.9	•
No Recommendation				3%

• Indicates that this product was recommended by less than 1% of pharmacists surveyed.
Bold type indicates the highest rating.

See also *Nausea; Vomiting*

THE ACTIVE INGREDIENT in Dramamine II (meclizine hydrochloride) doesn't cause drowsiness, which may be appealing to travelers who don't want to sleep through their vacation!

IN GENERAL, MOTION SICKNESS TREATMENTS are better at preventing illness than at curing it. If you have a history of motion sickness, be sure to start taking medication an hour or two before your departure time.

If you experience severe nausea and vomiting and your symptoms aren't relieved by over-the-counter medications, contact your doctor.

Muscle Pain

Muscle soreness that occurs as a result of overexertion in sports or other activities is caused by tiny tears in the muscle tissue. Muscle soreness isn't the same as a muscle spasm, which occurs when a muscle contracts and does not release. If possible, apply ice as soon as you're aware of the soreness, which will decrease not only the pain but also the chance of swelling. Gentle massage can also help alleviate pain. To avoid muscle injury, warm up with stretching exercises before working out.

SYMPTOMS: *Muscle stiffness, tightness or soreness in an area that was recently exerted*

INTERNAL PAIN RELIEVERS

| | Rated on a scale of 1 to 10 | | | Percentage Of Pharmacists Who Most Often Recommend |
	Most Effective	Speed Of Relief	Minimal Side Effects	
Advil	**8.7**	**8.1**	7.2	**51%**
Aleve	8.6	7.9	6.9	10%
Anacin Maximum Strength	7.9	7.8	7.0	•
Ascriptin Maximum Strength	7.8	7.8	7.2	•
Bayer Aspirin Extra Strength	8.0	7.9	7.1	2%
Bufferin Extra Strength	8.0	7.8	7.3	•
Ecotrin Maximum Strength	7.7	7.2	7.5	1%
Motrin IB	**8.7**	**8.1**	7.2	13%
Nuprin Pain Relief Formula	**8.7**	**8.1**	7.2	1%
Orudis KT	8.4	7.8	6.9	6%
Tylenol	7.1	7.4	**8.6**	5%
No Recommendation				11%

• Indicates that this product was recommended by less than 1% of pharmacists surveyed.
Bold type indicates the highest rating.

TYLENOL OR GENERIC ACETAMINOPHEN is the safest over-the-counter product for pain relief. However, if your pain is not relieved or there is significant inflammation, try an anti-inflammatory medication such as aspirin, ibuprofen, naproxen, etc., but be sure to take these medications with food, to avoid upsetting your stomach.

IF YOU'RE TAKING OTHER MEDICATION, check with your pharmacist or doctor about possible interactions before you take any of these products.

ADVIL, NUPRIN, AND MOTRIN IB are identical products containing 200 mg of ibuprofen.

IF YOU HAVE A HISTORY OF PEPTIC ULCERS, bleeding disorders, kidney disease, or asthma, contact your doctor before taking an over-the-counter anti-inflammatory medication such as aspirin, ibuprofen, naproxen, etc.

GENERIC EQUIVALENTS are available for these products. They are less expensive and just as effective as the name brands.

EXTERNAL PAIN RELIEVERS

	Rated on a scale of 1 to 10			Percentage Of Pharmacists Who Most Often Recommend
	Most Effective	Speed Of Relief	Minimal Side Effects	
Absorbine Jr. Extra Strength Liniment	7.1	7.6	7.7	•
Aspercreme	7.2	7.3	**8.1**	10%
BenGay Original Formula	7.5	7.8	7.8	11%
Capzasin-P	**8.0**	7.0	7.2	20%
Flex-All 454 Maximum Strength	7.8	**8.0**	**8.1**	**25%**
Heet Pain Relieving Liniment	7.5	**8.0**	7.5	1%
Icy Hot	7.7	7.9	7.8	7%
Thera-Gesic Extra Strength	7.9	**8.0**	7.7	4%
Therapeutic Mineral Ice	7.5	7.9	7.9	8%
No Recommendation				14%

• Indicates that this product was recommended by less than 1% of pharmacists surveyed.
Bold type indicates the highest rating.

continued on next page

MUSCLE PAIN CAUSED BY OVEREXERTION will almost always go away by itself in two or three days. Products that contain capsaicin, such as Capzasin-P, usually won't be appropriate for this kind of muscle pain, since they require one or two weeks of regular use to become effective.

ALL EXTERNAL ANALGESICS may cause irritation or burning and should not be used on broken or inflamed skin. Be sure to wash your hands thoroughly after using these products, and strictly avoid contact with the eyes or other mucous membranes such as your mouth, nostrils, and genitals. If excessive skin irritation occurs, stop using the product immediately.

IF YOU'RE USING AN EXTERNAL PAIN-RELIEVING RUB or cream, don't use a heating pad on the same area! Severe burns may occur.

Muscle pain that does not improve within one week of treatment using over-the-counter medicine should be evaluated by a doctor.

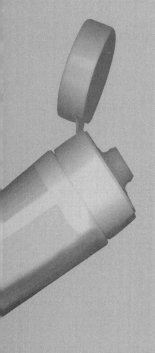

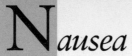ausea

Nausea, which is characterized by feelings of queasiness and an unsettled stomach, can be caused by a wide variety of different conditions. In general, a nauseous person should avoid motion and foods that will upset the stomach further. Sipping flat carbonated beverages and eating soda crackers may make some people feel better.

SYMPTOMS: *Queasiness • Upset Stomach*

	Rated on a scale of 1 to 10			Percentage Of Pharmacists Who Most Often Recommend
	Most Effective	Speed Of Relief	Minimal Side Effects	
Benadryl Allergy	5.5	5.6	5.4	4%
Bonine	7.3	6.9	6.8	6%
Calm-X	7.1	6.8	7.1	•
Dramamine Original Formula	7.4	6.9	6.4	7%
Emetrol	**8.0**	**8.1**	**8.9**	**67%**
Marezine	7.3	6.7	6.5	1%
Pepto-Bismol Maximum Strength	6.5	6.8	7.2	6%
No Recommendation				10%

• *Indicates that this product was recommended by less than 1% of pharmacists surveyed.*
Bold type indicates the highest rating.

Pharmacists Say...

PRODUCTS LIKE CALM-X AND EMETROL contain large amounts of glucose and fructose. If you have diabetes mellitus or a hereditary fructose intolerance, avoid these products.

PRODUCTS CONTAINING BISMUTH SUBSALICYLATE, such as Pepto-Bismol, contain salicylate. Because of the risk of Reye's Syndrome, these products should not be given to children who have chicken pox or the flu. They should also be avoided by anyone else who has been warned not to take aspirin or salicylates.

continued on next page

See also *Motion Sickness; Vomiting*

IF YOU HAVE GLAUCOMA, prostate disease, or breathing problems such as emphysema or chronic bronchitis, contact your pharmacist or doctor before taking any product containing an antihistamine. (Refer to Section Two, 'About the Products,' on page 131, for information on the active ingredients for the above products. Then see Section Three, the 'Glossary,' on page 175, for an explanation of those ingredients.)

See Your Doctor...

If your nausea persists for more than 48 hours or is associated with severe headache, abdominal pain, or chest pain, contact your doctor.

P*MS*

PMS refers to a group of symptoms that occur in the days prior to the onset of a period. This syndrome is most common in women in their 20s and 30s and is most likely related to hormonal changes, as it disappears during pregnancy and after menopause. You may be able to minimize the symptoms of PMS by avoiding fatty foods, salt, alcohol, and caffeine. Also exercise, plenty of rest, and avoidance of stress helps. These over-the-counter products are only for the treatment of menstrual cramps.

SYMPTOMS: *Weight gain • Fluid retention • Acne • Food cravings • Bloating • Breast tenderness • Fatigue • Headaches • Irritability • Mood swings • Difficulty in concentrating*

	Rated on a scale of 1 to 10			Percentage Of Pharmacists Who Most Often Recommend
	Most Effective	**Minimal Side Effects**	**Speed Of Relief**	
Advil	8.7	7.3	**8.2**	**43%**
Aleve	**8.8**	7.1	8.0	32%
Anacin Maximum Strength	7.1	7.2	7.5	•
Bufferin Extra Strength	7.0	7.2	7.4	•
Ecotrin Maximum Strength	6.7	7.3	6.7	•
Midol IB Cramp Relief Formula	8.7	7.3	8.1	5%
Motrin IB	**8.8**	7.3	**8.2**	10%
Nuprin Pain Relief Formula	**8.8**	7.3	**8.2**	2%
Tylenol	6.3	**8.4**	6.9	1%
No Recommendation				7%

• *Indicates that this product was recommended by less than 1% of pharmacists surveyed.*
Bold type indicates the highest rating.

Pharmacists Say...

TO AVOID CRAMPS AS MUCH AS POSSIBLE, your best bet is to start taking naproxen or ibuprofen a day or two before you expect your period to start. (Refer to Section Two, 'About the Products,' on page 131, for information on the active ingredients for the above products.)

continued on next page

ALEVE CONTAINS NAPROXEN, which is very similar to Anaprox, a prescription drug prescribed for cramps. However, it may cause the greatest gastrointestinal upset.

IF YOU HAVE A HISTORY OF PEPTIC ULCERS, bleeding disorders, kidney disease, or asthma, contact your doctor before taking an over-the-counter anti-inflammatory medication such as aspirin, ibuprofen, naproxen, etc.

ADVIL, NUPRIN, AND MOTRIN IB are identical products containing 200 mg of ibuprofen.

IF YOU ARE TAKING OTHER MEDICATION, check with your pharmacist or doctor about possible interactions before you take any of these products.

TAKE ANY ANTI-INFLAMMATORY MEDICATION such as aspirin, ibuprofen, naproxen, etc., with food to avoid upsetting your stomach.

FOR WATER RETENTION: Although there were a number of products included in the survey for water retention, none of the pharmacists found them to be effective, and they were not ranked or recommended.

GENERIC EQUIVALENTS are available for these products. They are less expensive and just as effective as the name brands.

See Your Doctor...

If your symptoms aren't relieved after using over-the-counter medications, contact your doctor.

Poison Ivy/Oak/Sumac

Poison ivy, oak, and sumac all contain the same chemical—uroshiol oil—which causes severe inflammatory response when it comes into contact with the skin. The oil can remain potent for years, so be sure to wash not only yourself with soap and water but also your clothes, shoes, and anything else such as gardening tools, doorknobs, pets, etc. In addition to the medications listed below, some people report that they feel better after using cool compresses or taking cool baths.

SYMPTOMS: *Itchy rash with small bumps and blisters*

	Rated on a scale of 1 to 10			Percentage Of Pharmacists Who Most Often Recommend
	Speed Of Relief	Most Effective	Desirable Duration Of Relief	
Aveeno Anti-itch Cream	7.7	7.7	6.7	10%
Benadryl Allergy	7.1	6.8	6.3	3%
Benadryl Itch Stopping Extra Strength	6.8	6.6	6.1	•
Caladryl	7.2	6.9	6.3	4%
Cortaid Maximum Strength	7.8	**8.1**	7.2	**23%**
Cortizone-10	7.7	7.9	7.1	20%
Dermoplast Pain Relieving Spray	8.1	7.2	6.3	2%
Ivarest 8-Hour Relief Medicated Cream	8.0	7.8	**7.5**	4%
Lanacort 10	7.6	7.9	7.2	•
Rhuli Gel	8.0	7.8	7.1	17%
Rhuli Spray	**8.2**	7.8	7.2	6%
Solarcaine Medicated First Aid	8.0	7.0	6.1	•
No Recommendation				13%

• *Indicates that this product was recommended by less than 1% of pharmacists surveyed.*
Bold type indicates the highest rating.

continued on next page

BE SURE TO KEEP the affected area clean and dry.

A GOOD WAY TO GET RELIEF is to take an oatmeal bath, gently pat the affected area dry, and apply a cream that contains a generic hydrocortisone 1 percent solution.

TAKING AN ORAL ANTIHISTAMINE such as Benadryl or its generic equivalent is more effective for this condition than using a topical cream. See 'General Warnings' (page xiii) regarding antihistamines.

HYDROCORTISONE PRODUCTS should not be applied to broken skin or used on large areas of the body.

THOROUGH BATHING WITH SOAP after exposure to poison ivy may prevent or lessen the outbreak.

See Your Doctor...

Severe cases or those that involve the face, eyes, or genitals should be seen by a doctor.

Ringworm

Like jock itch and yeast infections, ringworm can be caused by fungi that commonly live on the skin. When the skin's barrier is broken down by moisture and friction, it's prone to infection from these organisms. In addition to the medications listed below, it's important to keep the area dry, clean, and covered with loose clothing.

SYMPTOMS: *Round, red, raised lesions on the skin or scalp • Itching in the affected area*

	Rated on a scale of 1 to 10			Percentage Of Pharmacists Who Most Often Recommend
	Most Effective	**Speed Of Relief**	**Desirable Duration Of Relief**	
Lotrimin Antifungal AF	**9.1**	**7.6**	**8.3**	**70%**
Micatin	8.6	7.3	7.9	10%
Tinactin Antifungal	8.3	7.1	7.9	17%
Ting Antifungal	7.4	6.7	7.2	1%
No Recommendation				2%

Bold type indicates the highest rating.

Pharmacists Say...

RINGWORM IS STUBBORN and difficult to get rid of. Be sure to use the products exactly as directed, and continue treatment for one or two weeks after the symptoms are gone. If you stop using the product too soon, the condition may recur.

LOTRIMIN AF AND ITS GENERIC EQUIVALENTS cover a wider variety of fungi and yeasts than other products, so they may be more effective at ensuring that the condition is completely treated.

GENERIC EQUIVALENTS are available for these products. They are less expensive and just as effective as the name brands.

See Your Doctor...

If the affected area includes any part of your scalp, or if the condition doesn't clear up after two to three weeks of using over-the-counter medications, contact your doctor.

Sinus Congestion

Sinus congestion is a general term that refers to head congestion, with or without headaches, due to colds or allergies. If your symptoms are due to allergies, refer to the chart and tips on pages 6–7. If your symptoms are due to colds, refer to the charts and tips on page 30–33.

SYMPTOMS: *Head Congestion • Headache*

See Your Doctor...

If your congestion is associated with headache and a high fever or if your symptoms persist for more than one week, consult your doctor.

See also *Allergies; Colds; Congestion: Head*

Sore Throat

Sore throats may be a symptom of a viral or bacterial infection, or they may occur as a result of direct irritation from postnasal drip, excessive talking or shouting, or cigarette smoke. You might obtain relief by gargling with warm water or from lozenges.

SYMPTOMS: *Dry, red scratchy throat • Pain when swallowing*

For Adults

INTERNAL PAIN RELIEVERS

| | Rated on a scale of 1 to 10 | | | Percentage Of Pharmacists Who Most Often Recommend |
	Most Effective	Speed Of Relief	Minimal Side Effects	
Advil	7.8	7.5	6.9	28%
Aleve	7.5	7.1	6.7	3%
Anacin Maximum Strength	7.5	7.4	6.9	1%
Ascriptin Maximum Strength	7.5	7.3	7.0	•
Bayer Aspirin Extra Strength	7.6	7.5	6.8	7%
Bufferin Extra Strength	7.5	7.4	7.0	1%
Ecotrin Maximum Strength	7.3	6.7	7.1	2%
Motrin IB	**7.9**	**7.6**	7.0	5%
Nuprin Pain Relief Formula	7.8	**7.6**	6.9	1%
Orudis KT	7.4	7.2	6.6	2%
Tylenol	7.6	7.5	**8.6**	**39%**
No Recommendation				12%

• Indicates that this product was recommended by less than 1% of pharmacists surveyed.
Bold type indicates the highest rating.

continued on next page

PATIENTS MAY WANT to begin with a generic acetaminophen product, because of its relatively safe side effect profile.

ADVIL, NUPRIN, AND MOTRIN IB are identical products containing 200 mg of ibuprofen.

IF YOU ARE TAKING OTHER MEDICATION, check with your pharmacist or doctor about possible interactions before you take any of these products.

IF YOU HAVE A HISTORY OF PEPTIC ULCERS, bleeding disorders, kidney disease, or asthma, contact your doctor before taking an over-the-counter anti-inflammatory medication such as aspirin, ibuprofen, naproxen, etc.

TAKE ANY ANTI-INFLAMMATORY MEDICATION such as aspirin, ibuprofen, naproxen, etc., with food to avoid upsetting your stomach.

GENERIC EQUIVALENTS are available for these products. They are less expensive and just as effective as the name brands.

LOZENGES

	Rated on a scale of 1 to 10			Percentage Of Pharmacists Who Most Often Recommend
	Most Effective	Speed Of Relief	Minimal Side Effects	
Cepacol Maximum Strength Sore Throat Lozenges	8.1	8.3	8.8	11%
Cepastat Extra Strength Sore Throat Lozenges	**8.4**	**8.6**	**8.9**	28%
Fisherman's Friend Extra Strength	7.2	7.7	8.6	3%
Halls Menthol/Cough Suppressant Drops	6.9	7.6	8.7	2%
Ricola	6.9	7.5	8.8	2%
Spec-T Sore Throat Cough Suppressant Lozenges	8.2	**8.6**	8.8	15%
Sucrets Maximum Strength	7.8	8.2	8.8	7%
Vicks Chloraseptic Sore Throat Lozenges	8.3	8.5	8.8	**31%**
No Recommendation				1%

Bold type indicates the highest rating.

continued on next page

BEFORE YOU SPEND MONEY ON LOZENGES, try hard candy. If this doesn't help, and your sore throat is mild, you should use lozenges designed to simply soothe irritated throats. You should use only a lozenge that contains an anesthetic if you have a very severe sore throat.

TRY TO AVOID DRINKING LIQUIDS for a little while after finishing a lozenge so that you don't "wash away" the medicine from your throat.

IF YOUR SORE THROAT IS A RESULT OF POSTNASAL DRIP, consider taking a decongestant. See 'General Warnings' on (page xiii) regarding decongestants.

For Children

INTERNAL PAIN RELIEVERS

	Rated on a scale of 1 to 10			Percentage Of Pharmacists Who Most Often Recommend
	Most Effective	Minimal Side Effects	Speed Of Relief	
Advil Children's	8.3	6.9	**8.0**	5%
Motrin Children's	**8.4**	7.0	**8.0**	17%
Panadol Children's	7.9	8.3	7.8	•
Tempra 2	8.0	**8.6**	7.8	4%
Children's Tylenol	8.1	**8.6**	7.9	**68%**
No Recommendation				7%

• Indicates that this product was recommended by less than 1% of pharmacists surveyed.
Bold type indicates the highest rating.

BECAUSE ACETAMINOPHEN has fewer side effects, it is the treatment of choice for children.

BECAUSE OF THE RISK of Reye's Syndrome, don't give children any product that contains aspirin.

IF YOUR CHILD HAS A HISTORY of bleeding disorders, kidney disease, or asthma, contact your doctor before giving your child any product containing ibuprofen. (Refer to Section Two, 'About the Products,' on page 131, for information on the active ingredients for the above products.)

GENERIC EQUIVALENTS are available for these products. They are less expensive and just as effective as the name brands.

continued on next page

| | Rated on a scale of 1 to 10 | | | Percentage Of Pharmacists Who Most Often Recommend |
	Most Effective	Minimal Side Effects	Speed Of Relief	
Cepacol Regular Strength Sore Throat Lozenges	7.4	8.2	7.8	4%
Robitussin Cough Drops	6.8	8.3	7.5	4%
Sucrets Children's Sore Throat Lozenges	8.1	8.4	8.4	**42%**
Vicks Chloraseptic Sore Throat Lozenges	**8.3**	**8.5**	**8.9**	40%
No Recommendation				10%

Bold type indicates the highest rating.

Pharmacists Say...

BECAUSE OF THE RISK OF CHOKING, be very careful when giving lozenges to children. Do not let children run, play, or lie down with a lozenge in their mouth.

CHILDREN HAVE A TENDENCY TO SWALLOW COUGH DROPS and lozenges, which lessens their effectiveness at treating a sore throat.

BE SURE THAT THE CHILD doesn't use lozenges or sprays that contain an anesthetic within an hour or two before eating. A numb throat makes it easier for a child to choke on food.

See Your Doctor...

If you have a fever, swollen lymph nodes, or whitish patches on the back of your throat, or if your sore throat persists for more than one week, contact your doctor.

Sprains

Sprains occur when you stretch or tear a ligament. Ankles are the most commonly sprained joints, though wrists, shoulders, and other body parts can also suffer sprains. If you've sprained a joint, you should immediately apply ice and elevate the affected part of the body.

SYMPTOMS: *Pain and swelling in the affected joint*

	Most Effective	Speed Of Relief	Minimal Side Effects	Most Often Recommended
Advil	**8.7**	**8.1**	7.2	**53%**
Aleve	**8.7**	7.9	7.0	14%
Anacin Maximum Strength	7.8	7.7	7.1	•
Ascriptin Maximum Strength	7.8	7.6	7.2	•
Bayer Aspirin Extra Strength	7.9	7.7	7.0	3%
Bufferin Extra Strength	7.8	7.7	7.1	•
Ecotrin Maximum Strength	7.6	7.0	7.3	•
Motrin IB	**8.7**	**8.1**	7.2	11%
Nuprin Pain Relief Formula	**8.7**	**8.1**	7.2	1%
Orudis KT	8.6	7.8	7.0	5%
Tylenol Extra Strength	6.8	7.3	**8.7**	2%
No Recommendation				10%

Pharmacists Say...

TYLENOL OR GENERIC ACETAMINOPHEN is the safest over-the-counter product for pain relief. However, if your pain is not relieved or there is significant inflammation, try an anti-inflammatory medication such as aspirin, ibuprofen, naproxen, etc., but be sure to take these medications with food, to avoid upsetting your stomach.

IF YOU ARE TAKING OTHER MEDICATION, be sure to check with your pharmacist or doctor about possible drug interactions before you taking any of these products.

ADVIL, NUPRIN, AND MOTRIN IB are identical products containing 200 mg of ibuprofen.

continued on next page

IF YOU HAVE A HISTORY OF PEPTIC ULCERS, bleeding disorders, kidney disease, or asthma, contact your doctor before taking an over-the-counter anti-inflammatory medication such as aspirin, ibuprofen, naproxen, etc.

GENERIC EQUIVALENTS are available for these products. They are less expensive and just as effective as the name brands.

See Your Doctor...

If you experience an injury and the joint is swollen and discolored, won't support weight, and causes severe pain when moved, or if the pain does not improve within 72 hours, contact your doctor.

*S*unburn

Sunburn occurs from too much direct exposure to sunlight, resulting in a first-degree burn of the skin. (First-degree burns involve the outermost layers of skin, and are red and painful.) Sunburn is definitely linked with skin cancer, so your best bet is to avoid sunburn at all costs. Always wear sunscreen, avoid being in direct sun between 10 A.M. and 2 P.M., and wear long sleeves, sunglasses with UVA protection, and a hat when you're not swimming. If you do get burned, pain relievers such as aspirin can make you feel better; you might also apply an aloe moisturizer or take a cool bath to reduce the pain.

S Y M P T O M S : *Red, tender skin • Blisters*

TO RELIEVE PAIN

	Rated on a scale of 1 to 10			Percentage Of Pharmacists Who Most Often Recommend
	Most Effective	Speed Of Relief	Desirable Duration Of Relief	
Bactine First Aid	7.3	7.8	6.8	1%
Dermoplast Pain Relieving Spray	**8.7**	8.8	7.3	28%
Foille Medicated First Aid	8.1	8.4	7.2	10%
Lanacane Maximum Strength Spray Medication	8.3	8.6	7.4	8%
Solarcaine Medicated First Aid	8.6	**8.9**	**7.5**	**44%**
No Recommendation				10%

TO RELIEVE ITCHING

	Rated on a scale of 1 to 10			Percentage Of Pharmacists Who Most Often Recommend
	Most Effective	Speed Of Relief	Ease Of Use	
Cortaid Maximum Strength	**8.1**	**7.8**	**8.2**	**42%**
Cortizone-10	**8.1**	**7.8**	8.1	22%
No Recommendation				37%

Bold type indicates the highest rating.

continued on next page

See also *Burns*

TAKING ACETAMINOPHEN OR IBUPROFEN ORALLY can help relieve the general pain and discomfort associated with sunburn. See 'General Warnings' on (page xiii) regarding anti-inflammatory medications.

ITCHING AFTER A SUNBURN is usually caused by dry, damaged skin; applying a moisturizer between doses of a pain-relieving cream, spray, or lotion will keep the skin moist and relieve the itching as it heals.

CORTISONE PREPARATIONS are available as a cream, ointment, or lotion. Lotions cover larger areas, making them a better choice for sunburn.

If your skin is blistered, or if you experience confusion, weakness, lightheadedness, nausea, vomiting, or lethargy, contact your doctor.

Teething

About four to eight months after birth, a baby's teeth begin to push through the gums, causing pain, swelling, and irritation. Most babies like to use teething rings, which have the additional benefit of helping the teeth break through the gums when the baby bites down on it. Some teething rings can even be refrigerated so that the cool feeling helps alleviate the pain.

SYMPTOMS: *Increased drooling • Irritability*

	Most Effective	Speed Of Relief	Ease Of Use	Percentage Of Pharmacists Who Most Often Recommend
	Rated on a scale of 1 to 10			
Anbesol Baby Gel	8.4	**8.6**	**8.4**	28%
Babee Teething Lotion	8.0	8.2	8.2	•
Numz-it Gel Teething Pain Medication	8.1	8.4	8.2	1%
Orabase Baby	8.3	8.5	8.2	10%
Orajel Baby	**8.5**	**8.6**	**8.4**	**53%**
No Recommendation				9%

• *Indicates that this product was recommended by less than 1% of pharmacists surveyed.*
Bold type indicates the highest rating.

Pharmacists Say...

TYLENOL OR A GENERIC EQUIVALENT provides the best relief from teething pain. Products you apply to the gums will provide quick relief, but the effect won't last very long, as saliva will wash them away in less than half an hour.

THESE PRODUCTS SHOULD BE APPLIED very thinly to the gums. They contain benzocaine, which, if swallowed, could numb the throat. If the child shows any sign of irritation from these products, stop using them immediately.

MOST BABIES don't like the bitter taste of these products. A frozen teething ring works best.

See Your Doctor...

If your child doesn't respond to over-the-counter medications, you may wish to contact your doctor for advice.

Toothache

Toothaches are usually caused by bacteria and decay. If you have a toothache, see your dentist immediately and follow his or her recommendations for treatment. Until you get to the dentist, you can try taking a pain reliever such as aspirin, ibuprofen, or acetaminophen. Avoid hot foods and liquids, which can make the pain feel worse.

SYMPTOMS: *Throbbing, painful tooth • Pain when chewing • Pain at extremes of hot or cold*

INTERNAL PAIN RELIEVERS

	Rated on a scale of 1 to 10			Percentage Of Pharmacists Who Most Often Recommend
	Most Effective	**Speed Of Relief**	**Minimal Side Effects**	
Advil	**8.7**	8.0	7.2	**50%**
Aleve	8.4	7.7	7.0	7%
Anacin Maximum Strength	7.8	7.7	7.0	1%
Ascriptin Maximum Strength	7.8	7.6	7.0	•
Bayer Aspirin Extra Strength	7.9	7.7	6.9	2%
Bufferin Extra Strength	7.8	7.6	7.0	•
Ecotrin Maximum Strength	7.5	6.9	7.2	•
Motrin IB	**8.7**	8.0	7.3	14%
Nuprin Pain Relief Formula	**8.7**	**8.1**	7.3	1%
Orudis KT	8.2	7.5	6.9	3%
Tylenol	7.2	7.3	**8.5**	10%
No Recommendation				13%

• Indicates that this product was recommended by less than 1% of pharmacists surveyed.

Bold type indicates the highest rating.

	Rated on a scale of 1 to 10			Percentage Of Pharmacists Who Most Often Recommend
	Most Effective	Speed Of Relief	Ease Of Use	
Anbesol Maximum Strength Liquid	**8.2**	8.2	8.5	34%
Dent's Maxi-Strength Toothache Treatment	7.7	7.9	7.8	3%
Orajel Maximum Strength	**8.2**	**8.3**	**8.6**	**40%**
Red Cross Toothache Medication	7.8	7.8	7.7	10%
No Recommendation				12%

Bold type indicates the highest rating.

Pharmacists Say...

MEDICATIONS THAT YOU APPLY directly to the affected area don't provide relief that lasts very long. You should take an internal pain reliever like acetaminophen for longer relief.

DON'T EAT OR DRINK FOR ONE HOUR after using topical anesthetics, because swallowing may be impaired.

IF YOU ARE TAKING OTHER MEDICATION, check with your pharmacist or doctor about possible interactions before you take any of these products.

IF YOU HAVE A HISTORY OF PEPTIC ULCERS, bleeding disorders, kidney disease, or asthma, contact your doctor before taking an over-the-counter anti-inflammatory medication such as aspirin, ibuprofen, naproxen, etc.

ADVIL, NUPRIN, AND MOTRIN IB are identical products containing 200 mg of ibuprofen.

TAKE ANY ANTI-INFLAMMATORY MEDICATION such as aspirin, ibuprofen, naproxen, etc., with food to avoid upsetting your stomach.

GENERIC EQUIVALENTS are available for these products. They are less expensive and just as effective as the name brands.

See Your Doctor...

Always contact your dentist immediately for advice about a toothache.

Vaginal Dryness

Vaginal dryness can be caused by hormonal changes, infections, or the natural aging process. If you're experiencing dryness, be sure not to douche, which can make the problem worse.

SYMPTOMS: *Absence of normal vaginal moisture • Painful intercourse*

	Rated on a scale of 1 to 10			Percentage Of Pharmacists Who Most Often Recommend
	Most Effective	**Ease Of Use**	**Speed Of Relief**	
Gyne-Moistrin	8.6	8.2	8.7	9%
K-Y Jelly	8.3	7.7	8.5	30%
Lubricating Gel	8.2	7.9	8.5	2%
Moist Again	8.3	7.8	8.4	•
Replens	**8.8**	**8.4**	**8.8**	**57%**
No Recommendation				3%

• *Indicates that this product was recommended by less than 1% of pharmacists surveyed.*
Bold type indicates the highest rating.

Pharmacists Say...

REPLENS AND GYNE-MOISTRIN have applicators, which makes them easy to work with; however, they're quite expensive. K-Y Jelly is cheaper and just as effective.

CONVENIENCE AND EASE OF USE would be the main difference in these products.

See Your Doctor...

If you don't experience any relief after using over-the-counter medications, contact your doctor. In some cases, vaginal dryness in postmenopause women can indicate other health problems.

Vomiting

Vomiting is your body's response to an underlying illness. To give your stomach a chance to settle, don't eat or drink anything for at least an hour after vomiting. You should then start sipping clear liquids or flat soft drinks to keep from becoming dehydrated. When you're ready to eat again, stick to bland foods that are easily digested such as dry toast or crackers.

SYMPTOMS: *Vomiting • General weakness or sleepiness*

	Rated on a scale of 1 to 10			Percentage Of Pharmacists Who Most Often Recommend
	Most Effective	Speed Of Relief	Minimal Side Effects	
Benadryl Allergy	5.9	5.8	5.9	4%
Bonine	7.0	6.6	6.8	2%
Calm-X	6.7	6.6	7.2	•
Dramamine Original Formula	6.9	6.7	6.7	5%
Emetrol	**7.9**	**8.0**	**8.7**	**75%**
Marezine	6.9	6.5	6.6	•
Nauzene	6.9	6.5	6.3	•
Pepto-Bismol Maximum Strength	6.4	6.8	7.0	4%
No Recommendation				10%

• *Indicates that this product was recommended by less than 1% of pharmacists surveyed.*
Bold type indicates the highest rating.

continued on next page

See also *Motion Sickness; Nausea*

IF YOU CAN'T STOP VOMITING, oral medication may not be effective. Be sure that you don't become dehydrated, which is especially important for children and elderly people. To replenish fluids in your system drink an electrolyte replacement such as Pedialyte (for children) and Gatorade or other sports drinks (for adults).

PRODUCTS LIKE CALM-X AND EMETROL contain large amounts of glucose and fructose. If you have diabetes mellitus or a hereditary fructose intolerance, avoid these products.

PRODUCTS CONTAINING bismuth subsalicylate, such as Pepto-Bismol, contain salicylate and should also be avoided by anyone who has been warned not to take aspirin or salicylates.

IF YOU HAVE GLAUCOMA, prostate disease, or breathing problems such as emphysema or chronic bronchitis, contact your pharmacist or doctor before taking any product containing an antihistamine.

If you experience severe headache, abdominal pain, high fever, chills, or chest pain, or if the vomiting persists for more than one day, contact your doctor.

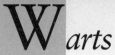

Warts

Warts are benign skin growths caused by a virus. They are contagious and occur on the hands and feet. If they occur on the botom of the feet, they are referred to as plantar warts and usually are painful.

SYMPTOMS: *Small, hard, skin-colored growths*

	Rated on a scale of 1 to 10			Percentage Of Pharmacists Who Most Often Recommend
	Most Effective	**Ease Of Use**	**Speed Of Relief**	
Compound W Wart Remover	8.0	7.7	6.8	17%
Dr. Scholl's Clear Away One Step Salicylic Acid Wart Remover	8.3	**8.1**	6.9	12%
DuoFilm Wart Remover	**8.5**	**8.1**	**7.1**	**49%**
DuoPlant Plantar Wart Remover	8.4	7.9	6.9	3%
Mediplast	8.4	7.6	**7.1**	13%
Wart-Off Wart Remover	8.0	7.6	6.6	4%
No Recommendation				2%

Bold type indicates the highest rating.

Pharmacists Say...

THESE PRODUCTS CONTAIN AN ACID that burns the skin. Be sure to apply these medications only to the affected area, not to any normal skin. You might want to apply a thin layer of petroleum jelly to the normal skin around the wart to protect it from the medication; however, be sure that you don't get any petroleum jelly on the wart itself.

BEFORE APPLYING THESE MEDICATIONS, soak the area to help soften it and remove dead tissue.

BECAUSE ALL OF THESE PRODUCTS USE THE SAME INGREDIENT (salicylic acid), they're equally effective; however, patches such as Dr. Scholl's Clear Away and Mediplast may be easier for you to work with than other forms of medication. Keep in mind that it can take several weeks of regular use before you see any results.

See Your Doctor...

If the warts do not respond after carefully using over-the-counter products for the period indicated, or if you have red or tender skin that extends beyond the area of treatment, contact your doctor.

Yeast Infection

Yeast infections are caused by the fungus *candida albicans,* which lives in the vagina at all times. Hormonal changes, antibiotics, spermicides, and diabetes can lead to changes in the vagina that promote the overgrowth of yeast. In addition to the medications listed below, eating yogurt may help restore the natural balance of the vagina.

SYMPTOMS: *Vaginal itching and burning • White vaginal discharge • Yeasty smell • Painful intercourse*

	Rated on a scale of 1 to 10			Percentage Of Pharmacists Who Most Often Recommend
	Most Effective	Ease Of Use	Speed Of Relief	
Femstat 3	**9.1**	**8.8**	**8.9**	**59%**
Gyne-Lotrimin 3	**9.1**	8.2	8.0	10%
Monistat 7	**9.1**	8.2	8.0	24%
Mycelex 7	**9.1**	8.2	8.0	2%
No Recommendation				5%

Bold type indicates the highest rating.

Pharmacists Say...

USE THESE PRODUCTS ONLY if you're sure you have a yeast infection and not some other kind of vaginal irritation. If you've never had a yeast infection before or are unsure of your symptoms, check with your doctor before using these medications.

IF THE PRODUCT YOU CHOOSE has a reusable applicator, be sure to wash it carefully with soap and hot water after each use. Otherwise, you run the risk of reinfecting yourself the next time you use the applicator.

MANY PEOPLE FIND that the prefilled applicators are the easiest to use.

THESE PRODUCTS SHOULD BE USED right before you go to bed, so that the medication stays in the vagina as long as possible without leaking out.

See Your Doctor...

If you're not sure whether or not you have a yeast infection, contact your doctor for a diagnosis. You should also contact your doctor if you have abdominal pain, fever, or a foul-smelling discharge, if your symptoms do not improve within three days, or if your symptoms recur within two months.

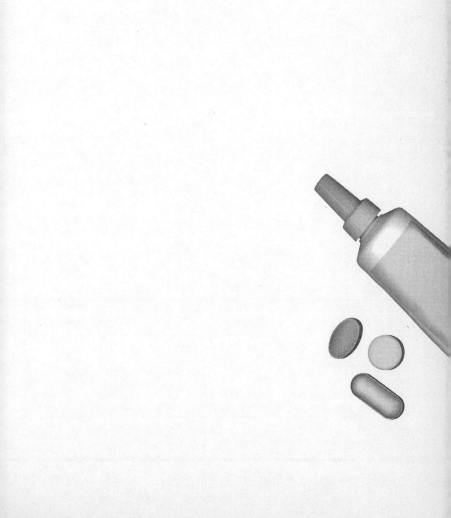

About the Products

This section provides an alphabetical listing of all the over-the-counter brands, their manufacturer, active ingredients, dosage form (tablet, capsule, liquid, etc.), and warnings.*

The following warnings apply to ALL of the drugs rated in this book. They have been listed here to reinforce their importance and to save space on the following pages. Although these and other specific warnings for each product are outlined for your reference, before taking any over-the-counter product read the label carefully and consult your pharmacist or doctor if you have any questions.

Use only as directed. Do not exceed the recommended dosage.

If you are pregnant or nursing a baby, seek the advice of a health-care professional before taking any over-the-counter product.

Keep all drugs out of reach of children.

In case of accidental overdose or ingestion, seek professional assistance or contact a poison control center immediately. Prompt medical attention is critical for adults as well as children even if you do not notice any signs or symptoms as a result of an overdose.

Also see 'General Warnings' at the front of this book on page xiii.

*Compiled as of September 1996.

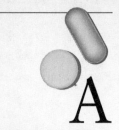

A

A AND D MEDICATED DIAPER RASH OINTMENT WITH ZINC OXIDE
Schering-Plough HealthCare Products

Dosage Form: ointment

Active Ingredients: white petrolatum, zinc oxide

Warning: No other warnings other than those listed at the beginning of this section have been indicated by the manufacturer.

A-200 LICE KILLING SHAMPOO
Hogil Pharmaceutical Corporation

Dosage Form: shampoo

Active Ingredients: piperonyl butoxide, pyrethrum extract

Warning: Use with caution on persons allergic to ragweed. For external use only. Do not use near the eyes or permit contact with mucous membranes, such as the nose, mouth or vagina, as irritation may occur. Keep out of the eyes when rinsing hair. *Adults and children:* Close eyes tightly and do not open until product is rinsed out. Also protect children's eyes with wash cloth, towel or other suitable material or by a similar method. If product gets into the eyes, immediately flush with water. If skin irritation or infection is present or develops, discontinue use and consult a doctor. Consult a doctor if infestation of eyebrows or eyelashes occurs.

ABSORBINE FOOT CARE ANTIFUNGAL
W. F. Young, Inc.

Dosage Form: liquid spray, cream

Active Ingredient: tolnaftate

Warning: For external use only. Use only as directed. Avoid contact with the eyes and mucous membranes. If skin redness or irritation develops, if condition worsens, or does not improve within 7 days, or clears up and occurs again within a few days, discontinue use and consult a doctor. Do not use on children under 2 years of age except under the advice and supervision of a doctor. Do not apply to wounds, or to damaged, broken (open) or irritated skin. Do not bandage tightly. Do not use with a heating pad.

ABSORBINE JR. EXTRA STRENGTH LINIMENT
W. F. Young, Inc.

Dosage Form: liquid

Active Ingredient: menthol

Warning: Use only as directed. Replace cap firmly. For external use only. If condition worsens, or symptoms persist for more than 7 days discontinue use and consult a doctor. Avoid contact with eyes. Do not use on children under 2 years of age except under the advice and supervi-

sion of a doctor. Do not apply to wounds or damaged skin. Do not bandage.

ACTIFED COLD & ALLERGY
Warner Lambert
Consumer Healthcare

Dosage Form: caplet, tablet

Active Ingredients: pseudoephedrine hydrochloride (HCl), triprolidine hydrochloride (HCl)

Warning: Do not exceed recommended dosage because at higher dosages, nervousness, dizziness, or sleeplessness may occur. If symptoms do not improve within 7 days or are accompanied by a fever, consult a doctor. Do not take this product if you have a breathing problem such as emphysema or chronic bronchitis, or if you have heart disease, high blood pressure, diabetes, thyroid disease, glaucoma or difficulty in urination due to enlargement of the prostate gland unless directed by a doctor. May cause excitability especially in children. May cause drowsiness; alcohol, sedatives, and tranquilizers may increase its drowsiness effect. Avoid alcoholic beverages while taking this product. Do not take this product if you are taking sedatives or tranquilizers without first consulting your doctor. Use caution while driving a motor vehicle or operating machinery. DRUG INTERACTION PRECAUTION: Do not use this product if you are now taking a prescription monoamine oxidase inhibitor (MAOI) (certain drugs for depression, psychiatric or emotional conditions, or Parkinson's disease) or for 2 weeks after stopping the MAOI drug. If you are uncertain if your prescription drug contains an MAOI, consult a health professional before taking this product.

ACTIFED COLD & SINUS
Warner Lambert
Consumer Healthcare

Dosage Form: caplet, tablet

Active Ingredients: pseudoephedrine hydrochloride (HCl), triprolidine hydrochloride (HCl), acetaminophen

Warning: Do not exceed recommended dosage because at higher dosages, nervousness, dizziness, or sleeplessness may occur. Do not take this product for more than 10 days. If symptoms do not improve or are accompanied by a fever that lasts for more than 3 days, or if new symptoms occur, consult a doctor. Do not take this product if you have a breathing problem such as emphysema or chronic bronchitis, or if you have heart disease, high blood pressure, diabetes, thyroid disease, glaucoma or difficulty in urination due to enlargement of the prostate gland unless directed by a doctor. May cause excitability especially in children. May cause drowsiness; alcohol, sedatives, and tranquilizers may increase its drowsiness effect. Avoid alcoholic beverages while taking this product. Do not take this product while taking sedatives or tranquilizers without first consulting your doctor. Use caution while driving a motor vehicle or operating machinery. Do not use with other products containing acetaminophen. DRUG INTERACTION PRECAUTION: Do not use this product if you are now

taking a prescription monoamine oxidase inhibitor (MAOI) (certain drugs for depression, psychiatric or emotional conditions, or Parkinson's disease) or for 2 weeks after stopping the MAOI drug. If you are uncertain if your prescription drug contains an MAOI, consult a health professional before taking this product.

ADVIL
Whitehall-Robins Healthcare

Dosage Form: caplet, tablet, gel caplet

Active Ingredient: ibuprofen

Warning: ASPIRIN SENSITIVE PATIENTS: Do not take this product if you have had a severe allergic reaction to aspirin, e.g.—asthma, swelling, shock or hives, because even though this product contains no aspirin or salicylates, cross-reactions may occur in patients allergic to aspirin. Do not take for pain for more than 10 days or for fever for more than 3 days unless directed by a doctor. If pain or fever persists or gets worse, if new symptoms occur, or if redness or swelling is present, consult a doctor. These could be signs of serious illness. If you are under a doctor's care for any serious condition, consult your doctor before taking this product. As with aspirin and acetaminophen, if you have any condition which requires you to take prescription drugs, or if you have had any problems or serious side effects from taking non-prescription pain relievers, do not take this product without first consulting your doctor. If you experience any symptoms which are unusual or seem unrelated to the condition for which you took this product, consult a doctor before taking any more of it. Although ibuprofen is indicated for the same conditions as aspirin and acetaminophen, it should not be taken with them except under a doctor's direction. Do not combine this product with any other ibuprofen-containing product.

ADVIL CHILDREN'S
Whitehall-Robins Healthcare

Dosage Form: liquid

Active Ingredient: ibuprofen

Warning: ASPIRIN SENSITIVE CHILDREN: This product contains no aspirin, but may cause a severe reaction to people allergic to aspirin. Do not use this product if your child has had an allergic reaction to aspirin, e.g.—asthma, swelling, shock or hives. *Call your doctor if:* your child is under a doctor's care for any serious condition or if taking any other drug. Your child has problems or serious side effects from using fever reducers or pain relievers. Your child does not get any relief within 1 day (24 hours) of treatment or if pain or fever gets worse. Redness or swelling is present in the painful area. If the sore throat is severe, lasts for more than 2 days, or occurs with fever, headache, rash, nausea or vomiting. Any new symptoms appear. *Do not use:* with any other product that contains ibuprofen, or any other pain reliever/fever reducer, unless directed by a doctor. For more than 3 days for fever or pain, unless directed by a doctor. For stomach pain, unless directed by a doctor. Your child is dehydrated (significant fluid loss) due to continued vomiting, diarrhea or lack of fluid intake. If imprinted plastic carton or bottle wrap is broken or missing.

ADVIL COLD & SINUS
Whitehall-Robins Healthcare

Dosage Form: caplet, tablet

Active Ingredients: pseudoephedrine hydrochloride (HCl), ibuprofen

Warning: ASPIRIN SENSITIVE PATIENTS: Do not take this product if you have had a severe allergic reaction to aspirin, e.g.—asthma, swelling, shock or hives, because even though this product contains no aspirin or salicylates, cross-reactions may occur in patients allergic to aspirin. Do not exceed recommended dosage because at higher dosages, nervousness, dizziness, or sleeplessness may occur. Do not take for colds for more than 7 days or for fever for more than 3 days unless directed by a doctor. If the cold or fever persists or gets worse, or if new symptoms occur, consult a doctor. These could be signs of serious illness. If you are under a doctor's care for any serious condition, consult a doctor before taking this product. As with aspirin and acetaminophen, if you have any condition which requires you to take prescription drugs or if you have had any problems or serious side effects from taking any non-prescription pain reliever, do not take this product without first discussing it with your doctor. If you experience any symptoms which are unusual or seem unrelated to the condition for which you took this product, consult a doctor before taking any more of it. Do not take this product if you have heart disease, high blood pressure, thyroid disease, diabetes or difficulty in urination due to enlargement of the prostate gland, unless directed by a doctor. Do not combine this product with other non-prescription pain relievers. Do not combine this product with any other ibuprofen-containing product. DRUG INTERACTION PRECAUTION: Do not use this product if you are now taking a prescription monoamine oxidase inhibitor (MAOI) (certain drugs for depression, psychiatric or emotional conditions, or Parkinson's disease) or for 2 weeks after stopping the MAOI drug. If you are uncertain if your prescription drug contains an MAOI, consult a health professional before taking this product. IT IS ESPECIALLY IMPORTANT NOT TO USE ASPIRIN DURING THE LAST 3 MONTHS OF PREGNANCY UNLESS SPECIFICALLY DIRECTED TO DO SO BY A DOCTOR BECAUSE IT MAY CAUSE PROBLEMS IN THE UNBORN CHILD OR COMPLICATIONS DURING DELIVERY.

AFRIN 12 HOUR NASAL
Schering-Plough HealthCare Products

Dosage Form: drops, pump spray, spray

Active Ingredient: oxymetazoline hydrochloride (HCl)

Warning: Do not exceed recommended dosage. This product may cause temporary discomfort, such as burning, stinging, sneezing, or an increase in nasal discharge. Do not use for more than 3 days. Use only as direct-ed. Frequent or prolonged use may cause nasal congestion to recur or worsen. If symptoms persist, consult a doctor. Do not take this product if you have heart disease, high blood pressure, thyroid disease, diabetes or difficulty in urination due to enlargement of the prostate gland unless directed by a doctor. Do not use this product on a child who has heart disease, high blood pressure, thyroid disease, or diabetes unless directed by a doctor. The use of this container by more than one person may spread infection.

AFRIN SALINE MIST
Schering-Plough HealthCare Products

Dosage Form: spray

Active Ingredient: sodium chloride

Warning: The use of this container by more than one person may spread infection.

AGORAL STIMULANT LAXATIVE
Warner Wellcome Consumer

Dosage Form: emulsion

Active Ingredients: phenolphthalein

Warning: Do not use laxative products when abdominal pain, nausea, or vomiting are present unless directed by a doctor. Laxative products should not be used for a period longer than 1 week unless directed by a doctor. If you have noticed a sudden change in bowel habits that persists over a period of 2 weeks, consult a doctor before using a laxative. Rectal bleeding or failure to have a bowel movement after use of a laxative may indicate a serious condition. Discontinue use and consult a doctor. If skin rash appears, do not use this product or any other preparation containing phenolphthalein.

ALEVE
The Procter & Gamble Company

Dosage Form: caplet, tablet

Active Ingredients: naproxen sodium

Warning: Do not take this product if you have had asthma, hives or any other severe allergic reaction after taking any pain reliever/fever reducer. Even though this product may not contain the same ingredient, Aleve could cause similar reactions in patients allergic to other pain relieving drugs. If you generally consume 3 or more alcohol-containing drinks per day, you should consult your doctor for advice on when and how you should take Aleve and other pain relievers. Do not take for pain for more than 10 days or for fever for more than 3 days unless directed by a doctor. Consult a doctor if: your pain or fever persists or gets worse; the painful area is red or swollen; you take any other drugs on a regular basis; you have had serious side effects from any pain reliever; you have any new or unusual symptoms; more than mild heartburn, upset stomach, or stomach pain occurs with use of this product or if even mild symptoms persist. Although naproxin sodium is indicated for the same conditions as aspirin, ibuprofen and acetaminophen, it should not be taken with them or other naproxen-containing products except under the direction of a doctor. IT IS ESPECIALLY IMPORTANT NOT TO USE ASPIRIN DURING THE LAST 3 MONTHS OF PREGNANCY UNLESS SPECIFICALLY DIRECTED TO DO SO BY A DOCTOR BECAUSE IT MAY CAUSE PROBLEMS IN THE UNBORN CHILD OR COMPLICATIONS DURING DELIVERY.

ALKA-SELTZER ORIGINAL
Bayer Corporation,
Consumer Care Division

Dosage Form: effervescent tablet

Active Ingredient: sodium bicarbonate

Warning: Children and teenagers should not use this medicine for chicken pox or flu symptoms before a doctor is consulted about Reye syndrome, a rare but serious illness reported to be associated with aspirin. Except under the advice and supervision of a doctor, do not take more than, ADULTS: 8 tablets in a 24 hour period, (60 years of age or older: 4 tablets in a 24-hour period), or use the maximum daily dosage for more than 10 days. Do not take this product if you are allergic to aspirin or have asthma, if you have bleeding problems, or if you are on a sodium restricted diet. If ringing in the ears or a loss of hearing occurs, consult a doctor before taking any more of this product. Do not take this product for more than 10 days unless directed by a doctor. If pain persists or gets worse, if new symptoms occur, or if redness or swelling is present, consult a doctor. These could be signs of a serious condition. DRUG INTERACTION PRECAUTION: If you are taking medicines for anticoagulation (thinning the blood), diabetes, gout or arthritis consult a doctor before taking this product. Antacids may interact with certain prescription drugs. If you are presently taking a prescription drug, do not take this product without checking with your doctor or health professional. IT IS ESPECIALLY IMPORTANT NOT TO USE ASPIRIN DURING THE LAST 3 MONTHS OF PREGNANCY UNLESS SPECIFICALLY DIRECTED TO DO SO BY A DOCTOR BECAUSE IT MAY CAUSE PROBLEMS IN THE UNBORN CHILD OR COMPLICATIONS DURING DELIVERY.

ALKA-SELTZER PLUS
COLD MEDICINE LIQUI-GELS
Bayer Corporation,
Consumer Care Division

Dosage Form: softgel

Active Ingredients: pseudoephedrine hydrochloride (HCl), chlorpheniramine maleate, acetaminophen

Warning: Do not exceed recommended dosage because at higher dosages, nervousness, dizziness, or sleeplessness may occur. Do not take this product for more than 7 days or for fever for more than 3 days unless directed by a doctor. If symptoms do not improve or are accompanied by a fever, consult a doctor. If sore throat is severe, persists for more than 2 days, is accompanied by or followed by fever, headache, nausea or vomiting, consult a doctor promptly. Do not take this product if you have a breathing problem such as emphysema or chronic bronchitis, or if you have heart disease, high blood pressure, diabetes, thyroid disease, glaucoma or difficulty in urination due to enlargement of the prostate gland unless directed by a doctor. May cause excitability especially in children. May cause drowsiness; alcohol, sedatives, and tranquilizers may increase its drowsiness effect. Avoid alcoholic beverages while taking this product. Do not take this product while taking sedatives or tranquilizers without first consulting your doctor. Use caution while driving a motor vehicle or operating machinery. Do not use with other products containing acetaminophen. DRUG INTERACTION PRECAUTION: Do not use this product if you are now taking a prescription drug for high blood pressure without first consulting your doctor or if you are now taking a prescription monoamine oxidase inhibitor (MAOI) (certain drugs for depression, psychiatric or emotional conditions, or Parkinson's disease) or for 2 weeks after stopping the MAOI drug. If you are uncertain if your prescription drug contains an MAOI, consult a health professional before taking this product.

AMERICAINE HEMORRHOIDAL OINTMENT
Ciba Self-Medication, Inc.*

Dosage Form: ointment

Active Ingredients: benzocaine

Warning: If condition worsens or pain persists for more than 7 days, or clears up and occurs again within a few days, discontinue use and consult a doctor. If the symptom being treated does not subside or if redness, irritation, swelling, pain or other symptoms develop or increase, discontinue use and consult a doctor. Do not exceed recommended dosage, unless directed by a doctor. In case of bleeding, consult a doctor promptly. Do not put this product into the rectum by using fingers or any mechanical device or applicator. Certain persons can develop allergic reactions to ingredients in this product. Do not use this product if you have a history of allergy to local anesthetics such as procaine, butacaine, benzocaine, or other "caine" anesthetics.

AMERICAINE TOPICAL ANESTHETIC
Ciba Self-Medication, Inc.*

Dosage Form: aerosol spray, ointment

Active Ingredient: benzocaine

Warning: For external use only. Avoid contact with the eyes. If condition worsens, if a rash or irritation develops, or if symptoms persist for more than 7 days or clears up and occur again within a few days, discontinue use of this product and consult a doctor. Certain persons can develop allergic reactions to ingredients in this product. Do not use this product if you have a history of allergy to local anesthetics such as procaine, butacaine, benzocaine, or other "caine" anesthetics. *For spray only:* Contents under pressure. Do not puncture or incinerate. Flammable mixture; do not use near fire or throw into fire. Do not store at temperatures above 49°C (120°F). Use only as directed. Intentional misuse by deliberately concentrating and inhaling the contents can be harmful or fatal.

ANACIN MAXIMUM STRENGTH
Whitehall-Robins Healthcare

Dosage Form: tablet

Active Ingredient: aspirin

Warning: Children and teenagers should not use this medicine for chicken pox or flu symptoms before a doctor is consulted about Reye Syndrome, a rare but serious illness reported to be associated with aspirin. If pain persists for more than 10 days, or redness or swelling is present, or in arthritic or rheumatic conditions affecting children under 12 years of age, consult a doctor immediately. These could be signs of serious illness. Do not take this product if you are allergic to aspirin, have asthma, have stomach problems (such as heartburn, upset stomach or stomach pain) that persist or recur, or if you have ulcers or bleeding problems, unless directed by a doctor. If ringing in the ears or loss of hearing occurs, consult a doctor before taking any more of this product. DRUG INTERACTION PRECAUTION: Do not take this product if you are taking a prescription drug for anticoagulation (thinning of blood), diabetes, gout or arthritis unless directed by a doctor. IT IS ESPECIALLY IMPORTANT NOT TO USE ASPIRIN DURING THE LAST 3 MONTHS OF PREGNANCY UNLESS SPECIFICALLY DIRECTED TO DO SO BY A DOCTOR BECAUSE IT MAY CAUSE PROBLEMS IN THE UNBORN CHILD OR COMPLICATIONS DURING DELIVERY.

ANBESOL BABY GEL
Whitehall-Robins Healthcare

Dosage Form: gel

Active Ingredient: benzocaine

Warning: Do not use this product for more than 7 days unless directed by a doctor or dentist. If sore mouth symptoms do not improve within 7 days, if irritation, pain or redness persists or worsens; or if swelling, rash or fever develops, see your doctor or dentist promptly. Do not exceed recommended dosage. Do not use this product if you have a history of allergy to local anesthetics such as procaine, butacaine, benzocaine, or other "caine" anesthetics. Fever and nasal congestion are not symptoms of teething and may indicate the presence of infection. If these symptoms persist, consult your doctor. Avoid contact with the eyes.

ANBESOL MAXIMUM STRENGTH
Whitehall-Robins Healthcare

Dosage Form: gel, liquid

Active Ingredient: benzocaine

Warning: Do not use this product for more than 7 days unless directed by a dentist or doctor. If sore mouth symptoms do not improve; if irritation, pain, redness, persists or worsens; or if swelling, rash or fever develops, see your dentist or doctor promptly. Do not exceed recommended dosage. Do not use this product if you have a history of allergy to local anesthetics such as procaine, butacaine, benzocaine, or other "caine" anesthetics. Avoid contact with the eyes. Extremely flammable. Keep away from fire or flame. Avoid smoking during application and until this product has dried.

ANUSOL HEMORRHOIDAL OINTMENT
Warner Wellcome Consumer

Dosage Form: ointment

Active Ingredients: pramoxine hydrochloride (HCl), zinc oxide, mineral oil

Warning: If condition worsens or does not improve within 7 days, consult a doctor. If the symptom being treated does not subside or if redness, irritation, swelling, pain or other symptoms develop or increase, discontinue use and consult a doctor. Do not exceed the recommended daily dosage unless directed by a doctor. In case of bleeding, consult a doctor immediately. Do not put this product into the rectum by using fingers or any mechanical device or applicator. Certain persons can develop allergic reactions to ingredients in this product.

AQUASITE
Ciba Vision Ophthalmics

Dosage Form: drops

Active Ingredients: polyethylene glycol, dextran 70

Warning: To avoid contamination do not touch tip of container to any surface. Replace cap after usage. If you experience eye pain, changes in vision, continued redness or irritation of the eye, or if the condition worsens or persists for more than 72 hours, discontinue use and consult a doctor. If you have glaucoma, do not use this product except under the advice and supervision of a doctor. Overuse of this product may produce increased redness of the eye. If the solution changes color or becomes cloudy, do not use.

ARTHRICARE TRIPLE MEDICATED PAIN RELIEVING RUB
Del Pharmaceuticals, Inc.

Dosage Form: cream

Active Ingredients: methyl salicylate, menthol, methyl nicotinate

Warning: For external use only. Use only as directed. Avoid contact with the eyes and mucous membranes. If skin redness or irritation develops, if condition worsens, or does not improve within 7 days, or clears up and occurs again within a few days, discontinue use and consult a doctor. If prone to allergic reaction to aspirin or salicylates, consult a doctor before using. Do not apply to wounds, or to damaged, broken (open) or irritated skin. Do not bandage tightly. Do not use with a heating pad, or immediately before or after taking a shower or bath. As part of its warming action temporary redness may occur.

ARTHRITIS HOT PAIN RELIEF CREME
Thompson Medical Company, Inc.

Dosage Form: cream

Active Ingredients: methyl salicylate, menthol

Warning: For external use only. Use only as directed. Avoid contact with the eyes and mucous membranes. If skin redness or irritation develops, if condition worsens, or does not improve within 7 days, or clears up and occurs again within a few days, discontinue use and consult a doctor. If prone to allergic reaction to aspirin or salicylates, consult a doctor before using. Do not use on children under 12 years of age. Do not apply to wounds, or to damaged, broken (open) or irritated skin. Do not bandage tightly. Do not use with a heating pad.

ASCRIPTIN MAXIMUM STRENGTH
Ciba Self-Medication, Inc.*

Dosage Form: caplet

Active Ingredient: aspirin

Warning: Children and teenagers should not use this medicine for chicken pox or flu symptoms before a doctor is consulted about Reye Syndrome, a rare but serious illness reported to be associated with aspirin. Do not take for pain for more than 10 days or for fever for more than 3 days unless directed by a doctor. If pain or fever persists or gets worse, if new symptoms occur, or if redness or swelling is present, consult a doctor. These could be signs of serious illness. Do not take this product if you are allergic to aspirin, have asthma, have stomach problems (such as heartburn, upset stomach or stomach pain) that persist or recur, or if you have kidney, ulcers or bleeding problems, unless directed by a doctor. If ringing in the ears or loss of hearing occurs, consult a doctor before taking any more of this product. DRUG INTERACTION PRECAUTION: Do not take this product if you are taking a prescription drug for anticoagulation (blood thinning), diabetes, gout, arthritis or a tetracycline antibiotic unless directed by a doctor. IT IS ESPECIALLY IMPORTANT NOT TO USE ASPIRIN DURING THE LAST 3 MONTHS OF PREGNANCY UNLESS SPECIFICALLY DIRECTED TO DO SO BY A DOCTOR BECAUSE IT MAY CAUSE PROBLEMS IN THE UNBORN CHILD OR COMPLICATIONS DURING DELIVERY.

ASPERCREME
Thompson Medical Company, Inc.

Dosage Form: cream, lotion

Active Ingredient: salycin

Warning: For external use only. Use only as directed. Avoid contact with the eyes and mucous membranes. If skin redness or irritation develops, if condition worsens or pain persists for more than 7 days or clears up and occurs again within a few days, discontinue use and consult a doctor. If prone to allergic reaction to aspirin or salicylates, consult a doctor before using. Do not use on children under 10 years of age. Do not apply to wounds, or to damaged, broken (open) or irritated skin

AURO-DRI EAR DROPS
Del Pharmaceuticals, Inc.

Dosage Form: drops

Active Ingredient: isopropyl alcohol

Warning: Do not use if you have ear damage or discharge, ear pain, irritation or rash in the ear, or are dizzy; consult a doctor. Do not use if you have an injury or perforation (hole) of the ear drum or after ear surgery unless directed by a doctor. Avoid contact with the eyes. Discontinue use and consult a doctor if undue irritation or sensitivity occurs. Keep away from fire or flame. If excessive ear wax remains after use of this product, consult a doctor.

AVEENO ANTI-ITCH
Rydelle Laboratories

Dosage Form: cream, lotion

Active Ingredient: calamine, pramoxine hydrochloride (HCl), camphor

Warning: For external use only. Avoid contact with the eyes. If condition does not improve or recurs within 7 days, discontinue use, and consult a doctor.

AVEENO MOISTURIZING
Rydelle Laboratories

Dosage Form: cream, lotion

Active Ingredient: colloidal oatmeal

Warning: No warnings have been indicated by the manufacturer.

AYR NON-MEDICATED SALINE
B. F. Ascher & Company, Inc.

Dosage Form: drops, spray, gel

Active Ingredient: sodium chloride

Warning: The use of this dispenser by more than one person may spread infection.

B

BABEE TEETHING LOTION
S.S.S. Company

Dosage Form: lotion

Active Ingredients: benzocaine, cetalkonium chloride

Warning: If sore mouth symptoms do not improve within 7 days, see your children's doctor or dentist promptly. Do not use this product if you have a history of allergy to local anesthetics such as procaine, butacaine, benzocaine, or other "caine" anesthetics.

BACIGUENT
Roberts Pharmaceutical Corporation

Dosage Form: ointment

Active Ingredient: bacitracin

Warning: For external use only. Do not use in the eyes or apply over large areas of the body. In case of deep or puncture wounds, animal bites or serious burns, consult a doctor. If the condition persists or gets worse, discontinue use and consult a doctor. Do not use longer than 1 week unless directed by a doctor.

BACKACHE MAXIMUM STRENGTH RELIEF
Bristol-Myers Products

Dosage Form: caplet

Active Ingredient: magnesium salicylate tetrahydrate

Warning: Children and teenagers should not use this medicine for chicken pox or flu symptoms before a doctor is consulted about Reye Syndrome, a rare but serious illness reported to be associated with aspirin. Do not take for pain for more than 10 days unless directed by a doctor. If

pain or fever persists or gets worse, if new symptoms occur, or if redness or swelling is present, consult a doctor. These could be signs of serious illness. Do not take this product if you are allergic to salicylates (including aspirin), have asthma, have stomach problems (such as heartburn, upset stomach or stomach pain) that persist or recur, or if you have ulcers or bleeding problems, unless directed by a doctor. If ringing in the ears or loss of hearing occurs, consult a doctor before taking any more of this product. DRUG INTERACTION PRECAUTION: Do not take this product if you are taking a prescription drug for anticoagulation (thinning of blood), diabetes, gout or arthritis unless directed by a doctor. IT IS ESPECIALLY IMPORTANT NOT TO USE ASPIRIN DURING THE LAST 3 MONTHS OF PREGNANCY UNLESS SPECIFICALLY DIRECTED TO DO SO BY A DOCTOR BECAUSE IT MAY CAUSE PROBLEMS IN THE UNBORN CHILD OR COMPLICATIONS DURING DELIVERY.

BACTINE FIRST AID ANTISEPTIC
Bayer Corporation,
Consumer Care Division

Dosage Form: liquid, spray

Active Ingredients: lidocaine hydrochloride (HCl), benzalkonium chloride

Warning: For external use only. Do not use in the eyes or apply over large areas of the body. In case of deep or puncture wounds, animal bites, or serious burns, consult a doctor. Stop use and consult a doctor if the condition worsens or if symptoms persist for more than 7 days, or clear up and occur again within a few days. Do not use longer than 1 week unless directed by a doctor. Do not use in large quantities, particularly over raw surfaces or blistered areas.

BAYER ASPIRIN EXTRA STRENGTH
Bayer Corporation,
Consumer Care Division

Dosage Form: caplet, tablet

Active Ingredient: aspirin

Warning: Children and teenagers should not use this medicine for chicken pox or flu symptoms before a doctor is consulted about Reye Syndrome, a rare but serious illness reported to be associated with aspirin. Do not take for pain for more than 10 days or for fever for more than 3 days unless directed by a doctor. If pain or fever persists or gets worse, if new symptoms occur, or if redness or swelling is present, consult a doctor. These could be signs of serious illness. Do not take this product if you are allergic to aspirin, have asthma, have stomach problems (such as heartburn, upset stomach or stomach pain) that persist or recur, or if you have ulcers or bleeding problems unless directed by a doctor. If ringing in the ears or loss of hearing occurs, consult a doctor before taking any more of this product. DRUG INTERACTION PRECAUTION: Do not take this product if you are taking a prescription drug for anticoagulation (thinning of blood), diabetes, gout or arthritis unless directed by a doctor. IT IS

ESPECIALLY IMPORTANT NOT TO USE ASPIRIN DURING THE LAST 3 MONTHS OF PREGNANCY UNLESS SPECIFICALLY DIRECTED TO DO SO BY A DOCTOR BECAUSE IT MAY CAUSE PROBLEMS IN THE UNBORN CHILD OR COMPLICATIONS DURING DELIVERY.

BEANO
AkPharma, Inc.

Dosage Form: tablet

Active Ingredient: alpha-galactosidase (enzyme)

Warning: Beano is made from safe, food-grade mold, however if a rare sensitivity occurs with allergic type symptoms, discontinue use. Galactosemics consult your doctor.

BENGAY ARTHRITIS FORMULA
Pfizer Inc., Consumer Care Group

Dosage Form: cream

Active Ingredients: methyl salicylate, menthol

Warning: For external use only. Use only as directed. Do not swallow. If swallowed, induce vomiting and call a doctor immediately. Avoid contact with eyes and mucous membranes. If skin redness or irritation develops, pain lasts for more than 10 days, or with arthritis-like conditions in children under 12, do not use and call a doctor. If prone to allergic reaction to aspirin or salicylates, consult a doctor before using. Do not apply to wounds, or to damaged, broken (open) or irritated skin. Do not bandage tightly. Do not use with a heating pad.

BENGAY ORIGINAL FORMULA
Pfizer Inc., Consumer Care Group

Dosage Form: ointment

Active Ingredients: methyl salicylate, menthol

Warning: For external use only. Use only as directed. Do not swallow. If swallowed induce vomiting and call a doctor. Avoid contact with eyes and mucous membranes. If skin redness or irritation develops, pain lasts for more than 10 days, or with arthritis-like conditions in children under 12, do not use and call a doctor. If prone to allergic reaction to aspirin or salicylates, consult a doctor before using. Do not apply to wounds, or to damaged, broken (open) or irritated skin. Do not bandage tightly. Keep away from eyes, mucous membranes, broken or irritated skin.

BENADRYL ALLERGY
Warner Lambert
Consumer Healthcare

Dosage Form: liquid, capsule, tablet, chewable tablet

Active Ingredient: diphenhydramine hydrochloride (HCl)

Warning: May cause excitability especially in children. Do not take this product unless directed by a doctor, if you have a breathing problem such as emphysema or chronic bronchitis, or if you have glaucoma, or difficulty in urination due to enlargement of the prostate gland. May cause marked drowsiness; alcohol, sedatives and tranquilizers may increase the drowsiness effect. Avoid alcoholic beverages

while taking this product. Do not take this product if you are taking sedatives or tranquilizers without first consulting your doctor. Use caution when driving a motor vehicle, operating machinery. Do not use any other products containing diphenhydramine while using this product.

BENADRYL ALLERGY DECONGESTANT
Warner Lambert
Consumer Healthcare

Dosage Form: liquid, tablet

Active Ingredients: pseudoephedrine hydrochloride (HCl), diphenhydramine hydrochloride (HCl)

Warning: Do not exceed recommended dosage because at higher dosages, nervousness, dizziness, or sleeplessness may occur. If symptoms do not improve within 7 days or are accompanied by a fever, consult a doctor. Do not take this product if you have a breathing problem such as emphysema or chronic bronchitis, or if you have heart disease, high blood pressure, diabetes, thyroid disease, glaucoma or difficulty in urination due to enlargement of the prostate gland unless directed by a doctor. May cause excitability especially in children. May cause drowsiness; alcohol, sedatives, and tranquilizers may increase its drowsiness effect. Avoid alcoholic beverages while taking this product. Do not take this product if you are taking sedatives or tranquilizers without first consulting your doctor. Use caution while driving a motor vehicle or operating machinery. Do not use any other products containing diphenhydramine while using this product. DRUG INTERACTION PRECAUTION: Do not use this product if you are now taking a prescription monoamine oxidase inhibitor (MAOI) (certain drugs for depression, psychiatric or emotional conditions, or Parkinson's disease) or for 2 weeks after stopping the MAOI drug. If you are uncertain if your prescription drug contains an MAOI, consult a health professional before taking this product.

BENADRYL ALLERGY/COLD
Warner Lambert
Consumer Healthcare

Dosage Form: tablet

Active Ingredients: pseudoephedrine hydrochloride (HCl), diphenhydramine hydrochloride (HCl), acetaminophen

Warning: Do not exceed recommended dosage because at higher dosages, nervousness, dizziness, or sleeplessness may occur. Do not take this product for more than 10 days. If symptoms do not improve or are accompanied by a fever that lasts for more than 3 days, or if new symptoms occur, consult a doctor. If sore throat is severe, persists for more than 2 days, is accompanied by or followed by fever, headache, rash, nausea or vomiting, consult a doctor promptly. Do not take this product if you have a breathing problem such as emphysema or chronic bronchitis, or if you have heart disease, high blood pressure, diabetes, thyroid disease, glaucoma or difficulty in urination due to enlargement of the prostate gland unless directed by a doctor. May cause excitability especially in children. May cause drowsiness; alcohol, sedatives, and tranquilizers

may increase its drowsiness effect. Avoid alcoholic beverages while taking this product. Do not take this product while taking sedatives or tranquilizers without first consulting your doctor. Use caution while driving a motor vehicle or operating machinery. Do not use with any other products containing diphenhydramine while using this product. Do not use with other products containing acetaminophen. DRUG INTERACTION PRECAUTION: Do not use this product if you are now taking a prescription drug for high blood pressure without first consulting your doctor or if you are now taking a prescription monoamine oxidase inhibitor (MAOI) (certain drugs for depression, psychiatric or emotional conditions, or Parkinson's disease) or for 2 weeks after stopping the MAOI drug. If you are uncertain if your prescription drug contains an MAOI, consult a health professional before taking this product.

BENADRYL ITCH STOPPING EXTRA STRENGTH
Warner Lambert
Consumer Healthcare

Dosage Form: cream, spray, gel, stick

Active Ingredient: diphenhydramine hydrochloride (HCl)

Warning: For external use only. Avoid contact with the eyes. If condition worsens, does not improve within 7 days, or if symptoms persist for more than 7 days or clear up and occur again within a few days, discontinue use and consult a doctor. Do not use on chicken pox, measles, blisters or on extensive areas of skin, except as directed by a doctor. Do not use on children under 12 years of age without consulting a doctor. Do not use with any other drugs containing diphenhydramine while using this product.

BENYLIN ADULT FORMULA
Warner Wellcome Consumer

Dosage Form: liquid

Active Ingredient: dextromethorphan hydrobromide

Warning: A persistent cough may be a sign of a serious condition. If cough persists for more than 1 week, tends to recur, or is accompanied by a fever, rash, or persistent headache consult a doctor. Do not take this product for persistent or chronic cough such as occurs with smoking, asthma, chronic bronchitis, emphysema, or if cough is accompanied by excessive phlegm (mucous) unless directed by a doctor. DRUG INTERACTION PRECAUTION: Do not use this product if you are now taking a prescription monoamine oxidase inhibitor (MAOI) (certain drugs for depression, psychiatric or emotional conditions, or Parkinson's disease) or for 2 weeks after stopping the MAOI drug. If you are uncertain if your prescription drug contains an MAOI, consult a health professional before taking this product.

BENYLIN COUGH SUPPRESSANT EXPECTORANT
Warner Wellcome Consumer

Dosage Form: liquid

Active Ingredients: guaifenesin, dextromethorphan hydrobromide

Warning: A persistent cough may be a

sign of a serious condition. If cough persists for more than 1 week, tends to recur, or is accompanied by a fever, rash or persistent headache, consult a doctor. Do not take this product for persistent or chronic cough such as occurs with smoking, asthma, chronic bronchitis, or emphysema, or where cough is accompanied by excessive phlegm (mucous) unless directed by a doctor. DRUG INTERACTION PRECAUTION: Do not use this product if you are now taking a prescription monoamine oxidase inhibitor (MAOI) (certain drugs for depression, psychiatric or emotional conditions, or Parkinson's disease) or for 2 weeks after stopping the MAOI drug. If you are uncertain if your prescription drug contains an MAOI, consult a health professional before taking this product.

BENYLIN MULTI-SYMPTOM
Warner Wellcome Consumer

Dosage Form: liquid

Active Ingredients: pseudoephedrine hydrochloride (HCl), guaifenesin, dextromethorphan hydrobromide

Warning: Do not exceed recommended dosage because at higher dosages, nervousness, dizziness, or sleeplessness may occur. If symptoms do not improve within 7 days or are accompanied by a fever, consult a doctor. Do not take this product if you have heart disease, high blood pressure, thyroid disease, diabetes, or difficulty in urination due to enlargement of the prostate gland unless directed by a doctor. A persistent cough may be a sign of a serious condition. If cough persists for more than 1 week, tends to recur, or is accompanied by a fever, rash or persistent headache, consult a doctor. Do not take this product for persistent or chronic cough such as occurs with smoking, asthma, chronic bronchitis, or emphysema, or where cough is accompanied by excessive phlegm (mucous) unless directed by a doctor. DRUG INTERACTION PRECAUTION: Do not use this product if you are now taking a prescription monoamine oxidase inhibitor (MAOI) (certain drugs for depression, psychiatric or emotional conditions, or Parkinson's disease) or for 2 weeks after stopping the MAOI drug. If you are uncertain if your prescription drug contains an MAOI, consult a health professional before taking this product.

BENYLIN PEDIATRIC
Warner Wellcome Consumer

Dosage Form: liquid

Active Ingredient: dextromethorphan hydrobromide

Warning: A persistent cough may be a sign of a serious condition. If cough persists for more than 1 week, tends to recur, or is accompanied by a fever, rash, or persistent headache consult a doctor. Do not take this product for persistent or chronic cough such as occurs with smoking, asthma, chronic bronchitis, emphysema, or if cough is accompanied by excessive phlegm (mucous) unless directed by a doctor. Do not take this product if you are hypersensitive to any of its ingredients. DRUG INTERACTION PRECAUTION: Do not use this product if you are now taking a prescription monoamine oxidase inhibitor (MAOI) (certain

drugs for depression, psychiatric or emotional conditions, or Parkinson's disease) or for 2 weeks after stopping the MAOI drug. If you are uncertain if your prescription drug contains an MAOI, consult a health professional before taking this product.

BETADINE SOLUTION
The Purdue Frederick Company

Dosage Form: solution

Active Ingredient: povidone-iodine

Warning: For external use only. In case of deep or puncture wounds or serious burns, consult a doctor. If redness, irritation, swelling or pain persists or increases, or if infection occurs, discontinue use and consult a doctor.

BLISTEX LIP MEDEX
Blistex Inc.

Dosage Form: ointment

Active Ingredients: petrolatum, camphor, menthol, phenol

Warning: For children under 2 years old, consult a doctor. If condition worsens or symptoms persist consult a doctor.

BLISTEX MEDICATED LIP BALM
Blistex Inc.

Dosage Form: stick

Active Ingredients: padimate O, oxybenzone, dimethicone

Warning: For external use only. Avoid direct contact with the eyes. If contact occurs, rinse thoroughly with water. Discontinue use if signs of irritation or rash occur. If irritation or rash persists, consult a doctor. As with all personal care items, this product should be used by one individual only.

BLISTEX MEDICATED LIP OINTMENT
Blistex Inc.

Dosage Form: ointment

Active Ingredients: allantoin, menthol, camphor, phenol

Warning: For external use only. Avoid direct contact with the eyes. If condition worsens or symptoms persist for more than 7 days, or clear up and occur again within a few days, discontinue use and consult a doctor. Do not apply over large areas of the body. As with all products, a few individuals may be sensitive or allergic to this formula. As with all personal care items, this product should be used by one individual only.

BOIL EASE
Del Pharmaceuticals, Inc.

Dosage Form: ointment

Active Ingredients: benzocaine

Warning: For external use only. Avoid contact with the eyes. Do not use on boils on the lips, nose, cheeks, or forehead. Consult a doctor for treatment of boils on those areas. If condition worsens, or does not improve, fever occurs, redness around a boil develops, consult a doctor. Do not use this product for more than 7 days. Certain persons can develop allergic reactions to ingredients in this product. Do not use this product if you have a history of allergy to local anesthetics such as procaine, butacaine, benzocaine, or other "caine" anesthetics.

BONINE
Pfizer Inc., Consumer Care Group

Dosage Form: chewable tablet

Active Ingredient: meclizine hydrochloride (HCl)

Warning: Do not give to children under 12 years of age unless directed by a doctor. Do not take this product, if you have breathing problems such as emphysema, or chronic bronchitis, or if you have glaucoma, or difficulty in urination due to enlargement of the prostate gland, unless directed by a doctor. May cause drowsiness; alcohol, sedatives, and tranquilizers may increase its drowsiness effect. Avoid alcoholic beverages while taking this product. Do not take this product if you are taking sedatives or tranquilizers without first consulting your doctor. Do not drive or operate dangerous machinery while taking this medication. Not for frequent or prolonged use, except on advice of a doctor. Do not exceed recommended dosage.

BUFFERIN ARTHRITIS STRENGTH
Bristol-Myers Products

Dosage Form: caplet

Active Ingredient: aspirin

Warning: Children and teenagers should not use this medicine for chicken pox or flu symptoms before a doctor is consulted about Reye Syndrome, a rare but serious illness reported to be associated with aspirin. Do not take for pain for more than 10 days or for fever for more than 3 days unless directed by a doctor. If pain or fever persists or gets worse, if new symptoms occur, or if redness or swelling is present, consult a doctor. These could be signs of serious illness. Do not take this product if you are allergic to aspirin, have asthma, have stomach problems (such as heartburn, upset stomach or stomach pain) that persist or recur, or if you have ulcers or bleeding problems, unless directed by a doctor. If ringing in the ears or loss of hearing occurs, consult a doctor before taking any more of this product. DRUG INTERACTION PRECAUTION: Do not take this product if you are taking a prescription drug for anticoagulation (thinning of blood), diabetes, gout or arthritis unless directed by a doctor. IT IS ESPECIALLY IMPORTANT NOT TO USE ASPIRIN DURING THE LAST 3 MONTHS OF PREGNANCY UNLESS SPECIFICALLY DIRECTED TO DO SO BY A DOCTOR BECAUSE IT MAY CAUSE PROBLEMS IN THE UNBORN CHILD OR COMPLICATIONS DURING DELIVERY.

BUFFERIN EXTRA STRENGTH
Bristol-Myers Products

Dosage Form: tablet

Active Ingredient: aspirin

Warning: Children and teenagers should not use this medicine for chicken pox or flu symptoms before a doctor is consulted about Reye Syndrome, a rare but serious illness reported to be associated with aspirin. Do not take for pain for more than 10 days or for fever for more than 3 days unless directed by a doctor. If pain or fever persists or gets worse, if new symptoms occur, or if redness or swelling is present, consult a doctor. These could be signs of serious illness. Do not take this product if you are allergic to aspirin, have asthma, have stomach problems (such as heartburn, upset stomach or stomach pain) that persist or recur, or if you have ulcers or bleeding problems, unless directed by a doctor. If ringing in the ears or loss of hearing occurs, consult a doctor before taking any more of this product. DRUG INTERACTION PRECAUTION: Do not take this product if you are taking a prescription drug for anticoagulation (thinning of blood), diabetes, gout or arthritis unless directed by a doctor. IT IS ESPECIALLY IMPORTANT NOT TO USE ASPIRIN DURING THE LAST 3 MONTHS OF PREGNANCY UNLESS SPECIFICALLY DIRECTED TO DO SO BY A DOCTOR BECAUSE IT MAY CAUSE PROBLEMS IN THE UNBORN CHILD OR COMPLICATIONS DURING DELIVERY.

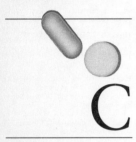

C

CALADRYL
Warner Wellcome Consumer

Dosage Form: lotion

Active Ingredients: pramoxine hydrochloride (HCl), calamine

Warning: For external use only. Avoid contact with the eyes. If condition worsens, does not improve, or if symptoms persist for more than 7 days or clear up and occur again within a few days, discontinue use of this product and consult a doctor.

CALM-X
Republic Drug Company, Inc.

Dosage Form: tablet

Active Ingredient: dimenhydrinate

Warning: Do not give to children under 2 years of age unless directed by a doctor. Do not take this product, unless directed by a doctor, if you have breathing problems such as emphysema, or chronic bronchitis, or if you have glaucoma, or difficulty in urination due to enlargement of the prostate gland. May cause marked drowsiness: alcohol, sedatives, and tranquilizers may increase its drowsiness effect. Avoid alcoholic beverages while taking this product. Do not take this product if you are taking sedatives or tranquilizers, without first consulting your doctor. Use caution when driving a motor vehicle or operating machinery. Not for frequent or prolonged use, except on advice of a doctor. Do not exceed recommended dosage.

CAMPHO-PHENIQUE ORIGINAL COLD SORE GEL
Bayer Corporation, Consumer Care Division

Dosage Form: gel

Active Ingredients: camphor, phenol

Warning: For external use only. Do not use in or near the eyes or apply over large areas of the body. If product gets into the eyes, flush thoroughly with water and obtain medical attention. Stop use and consult a doctor if condition worsens or if symptoms persist for more than 7 days or clear up and recur again within a few days. Do not use longer than a week unless directed by a doctor. Do not bandage. Do not induce vomiting in case of accidental ingestion.

CAMPHO-PHENIQUE PAIN RELIEVING ANTISEPTIC
Bayer Corporation, Consumer Care Division

Dosage Form: gel, liquid

Active Ingredients: camphor, phenol

Dosage Form: cream

Active Ingredients: bacitracin, zinc

Warning: For external use only. Do not use in or near the eyes or apply over large areas of the body. If product gets into the eyes, flush thoroughly with water and obtain medical attention. In case of deep or puncture wounds, animal bites, or serious burns, consult a doctor. Stop use and consult a doctor if condition worsens or symptoms persist for more than 7 days, or clear up and occur again within a few days. Do not use longer than a week unless directed by a doctor. Do not bandage. Do not induce vomiting in case of accidental ingestion.

CAPZASIN-P
Thompson Medical Company, Inc.

Dosage Form: cream

Active Ingredient: capsaicin

Warning: For external use only. Use only as directed. Transient burning may occur upon application, but generally disappears in several days. Avoid contact with eyes and mucous membranes. If skin redness or irritation develops, if condition worsens, or does not improve within 7 days, or clears up and occurs again within a few days, discontinue use and consult a doctor. Do not apply to wounds, or to damaged, broken (open) or irritated skin. Do not bandage tightly. Do not use with a heating pad.

CARMEX LIP BALM
Carma Laboratories, Inc.

Dosage Form: ointment

Active Ingredients: menthol, camphor, salicylic acid, phenol, alum

Warning: Use only as directed. As with all personal care items, this product should be used by one individual only.

CELLUVISC
Allergan, Inc.

Dosage Form: drops

Active Ingredient: carboxymethylcellulose sodium

Warning: To avoid contamination do not touch tip of container to any surface. Do not reuse. Once open, discard. If you experience eye pain, changes in vision, continued redness or irritation of the eye, or if the condition worsens or persists for more than 72 hours, discontinue use and consult a doctor. If you have glaucoma, do not use this product except under the

advice and supervision of a doctor. If the solution changes color or becomes cloudy, do not use.

CEPACOL MAXIMUM STRENGTH SORE THROAT LOZENGES
J. B. Williams Company, Inc.

Dosage Form: lozenge

Active Ingredients: benzocaine, menthol

Warning: If sore throat is severe, persists for more than 2 days, is accompanied or followed by a fever, headache, rash, swelling, nausea or vomiting, consult a doctor promptly. Certain persons can develop allergic reactions to ingredients in this product. Do not use this product if you have a history of allergy to local anesthetics such as procaine, butacaine, benzocaine, or other "caine" anesthetics. Do not administer to children under 6 years of age unless directed by a doctor.

CEPACOL REGULAR STRENGTH SORE THROAT LOZENGES
J. B. Williams Company, Inc.

Dosage Form: lozenge

Active Ingredient: menthol

Warning: If sore throat is severe, persists for more than 2 days, is accompanied or followed by a fever, headache, rash, swelling, nausea or vomiting, consult a doctor promptly. Do not administer to children under 6 years of age unless directed by a doctor.

CEPASTAT EXTRA STRENGTH SORE THROAT LOZENGES
SmithKline Beecham Consumer Health Care, L.P.

Dosage Form: lozenge

Active Ingredient: phenol

Warning: If sore throat is severe, persists for more than 2 days, is accompanied or followed by a fever, headache, rash, swelling, nausea or vomiting, consult a doctor promptly. If sore throat symptoms do not improve within 7 days, or if irritation, pain, or redness persists or worsens, see your dentist or doctor promptly. NOTE TO DIABETICS: Each lozenge contains approximately 8 calories from 2 grams of sorbitol.

CETAPHIL
Galderma Laboratories, Inc.

Dosage Form: bar

Active Ingredient: No active ingredients have been indicated by the manufacturer.

Warning: No warnings have been indicated by the manufacturer.

CHAPSTICK LIP BALM
Whitehall-Robins Healthcare

Dosage Form: stick

Active Ingredients: petrolatum, padimate O

Warning: As with all personal care items, this product should be used by one individual only.

CHAPSTICK SUNBLOCK 15
Whitehall-Robins Healthcare

Dosage Form: stick

Active Ingredients: white petrolatum, padimate O, oxybenzone

Warning: For external use only. Avoid contact with eyes. Discontinue use if signs of irritation or rash occur. As with all personal care items, this product should be used by one individual only.

CHARCOCAPS
Requa, Inc.

Dosage Form: caplets, capsules, tablets

Active Ingredients: activated charcoal

Warning: May absorb other medication (such as heart drugs or birth control) if taken at the same time. Consult with your doctor if taking medication as it may interfere with their effectiveness. It is suggested to allow at least 1 hour after or 2 hours before taking any medication. May cause darkening of the stool.*

This statement has not been evaluated by the Food and Drug Administration. This product is not intended to diagnose, treat, cure, or prevent any disease.

CHERACOL D COUGH FORMULA
Roberts Pharmaceutical Corporation

Dosage Form: liquid

Active Ingredients: guaifenesin, dextromethorphan hydrobromide

Warning: Do not give this product to children under 2 years of age unless under the advice and supervision of a doctor. A persistent cough may be a sign of a serious condition. If cough persists for more than 1 week, tends to recur, or is accompanied by a fever, rash or persistent headache, consult a doctor. Do not take this product for persistent or chronic cough such as occurs with smoking, asthma, chronic bronchitis, or emphysema, or where cough is accompanied by excessive phlegm (mucous) unless directed by a doctor. DRUG INTERACTION PRECAUTION: Do not use this product if you are now taking a prescription monoamine oxidase inhibitor (MAOI) (certain drugs for depression, psychiatric or emotional conditions, or Parkinson's disease) or for 2 weeks after stopping the MAOI drug. If you are uncertain if your prescription drug contains an MAOI, consult a health professional before taking this product.

CHLOR-TRIMETON ALLERGY
Schering-Plough HealthCare Products

Dosage Form: syrup

Active Ingredient: chlorpheniramine maleate

Warning: May cause excitability, especially in children. Do not take this product if you have asthma, glaucoma, emphysema, chronic pulmonary disease, shortness of breath, difficulty in breathing, or difficulty in urination due to enlargement of the prostate gland unless directed by a doctor. May cause drowsiness; alcohol, sedatives and tranquilizers may increase the drowsiness effect. Avoid alcoholic beverages while taking this product. Do not take this product if you are taking sedatives or tranquilizers without first consulting your doctor. Use caution while driving a motor vehicle or operating machinery.

CHLOR-TRIMETON ALLERGY 8 HOUR
Schering-Plough HealthCare Products

Dosage Form: tablet

Active Ingredient: chlorpheniramine maleate

Warning: May cause excitability, especially in children. Do not give this product to children under 12 years, except under the advice and supervision of a doctor. Do not take this product if you have asthma, glaucoma, emphysema, chronic pulmonary disease, shortness of breath, difficulty in breathing, or difficulty in urination due to enlargement of the prostate gland unless directed by a doctor. May cause drowsiness; alcohol, sedatives and tranquilizers may increase the drowsiness effect. Avoid alcoholic beverages while taking this product. Do not take this product if you are taking sedatives or tranquilizers without first consulting your doctor. Use caution while driving a motor vehicle or operating machinery. Do not crush or chew tablets. Swallow whole.

CHLOR-TRIMETON ALLERGY 12 HOUR
Schering-Plough HealthCare Products

Dosage Form: tablet

Active Ingredient: chlorpheniramine maleate

Warning: May cause excitability, especially in children. Do not give this product to children under 12 years, except under the advice and supervision of a doctor. Do not take this product if you have asthma, glaucoma, emphysema, chronic pulmonary disease, shortness of breath, difficulty in breathing, or difficulty in urination due to enlargement of the prostate gland unless directed by a doctor. May cause drowsiness; alcohol, sedatives and tranquilizers may increase the drowsiness effect. Avoid alcoholic beverages while taking this product. Do not take this product if you are taking sedatives or tranquilizers without first consulting your doctor. Use caution while driving a motor vehicle or operating machinery. Do not crush or chew tablets. Swallow whole.

CHLOR-TRIMETON ALLERGY DECONGESTANT 12 HOUR
Schering-Plough HealthCare Products

Dosage Form: tablet

Active Ingredients: pseudoephedrine sulfate, chlorpheniramine maleate

Warning: Do not exceed recommended dosage because at higher dosages, nervousness, dizziness, or sleeplessness may occur. Do not take for more than 7 days. If symptoms do not improve or are accompanied by a fever, consult a doctor. Do not take this product if you have a breathing problem such as emphysema or chronic bronchitis, or if you have heart disease, high blood pressure, diabetes, thyroid disease, glaucoma or difficulty in urination due to enlargement of the prostate gland, unless directed by a doctor. May cause excitability especially in children. May cause drowsiness; alcohol, sedatives, and tranquilizers may increase its drowsiness effect. Avoid alcoholic beverages while taking this product. Do not take this product if you are taking sedatives or tranquilizers without first consulting your doctor. Use caution while driving a motor vehicle or operating machinery. Do not use with other products containing acetaminophen. DRUG INTERACTION PRECAUTION: Do not use this product if you are now taking a prescription monoamine oxidase

inhibitor (MAOI) (certain drugs for depression, psychiatric or emotional conditions, or Parkinson's disease) or for 2 weeks after stopping the MAOI drug. If you are uncertain if your prescription drug contains an MAOI, consult a health professional before taking this product. Do not crush or chew tablets. Swallow whole.

CHLOR-TRIMETON ALLERGY SINUS HEADACHE
Schering-Plough HealthCare Products

Dosage Form: caplet

Active Ingredients: phenylpropanolamine hydrochloride (HCl), chlorpheniramine maleate, acetaminophen

Warning: Do not exceed recommended dosage because at higher dosages, nervousness, dizziness, or sleeplessness may occur. Do not take this product for pain or congestion for more than 7 days and do not take for fever for more than 3 days unless directed by a doctor. If pain or fever persists or gets worse, if new symptoms occur or if redness or swelling is persistent, consult a doctor because these could be signs of a serious condition. Do not take this product if you have a breathing problem such as emphysema or chronic bronchitis, or if you have heart disease, high blood pressure, diabetes, thyroid disease, glaucoma, or difficulty in urination due to enlargement of the prostate gland unless directed by a doctor. May cause excitability especially in children. May cause drowsiness; alcohol, sedatives, and tranquilizers may increase its drowsiness effect. Avoid alcoholic beverages while taking this product. Do not take this product if you are taking sedatives or tranquilizers without first consulting your doctor. Use caution while driving a motor vehicle or operating machinery. DRUG INTERACTION PRECAUTION: Do not use this product if you are now taking a prescription monoamine oxidase inhibitor (MAOI) (certain drugs for depression, psychiatric or emotional conditions, or Parkinson's disease) or for 2 weeks after stopping the MAOI drug. If you are uncertain if your prescription drug contains an MAOI, consult a health professional before taking this product. Do not take this product if you are taking an appetite-controlling medication containing phenylpropanolamine without first consulting your doctor. Do not use with other products containing acetaminophen.

CHLOR-TRIMETON NON-DROWSY NASAL DECONGESTANT 4 HOUR
Schering-Plough HealthCare Products

Dosage Form: tablet

Active Ingredient: pseudoephedrine sulfate

Warning: Do not exceed recommended dosage because at higher dosages, nervousness, dizziness, or sleeplessness may occur. If symptoms do not improve within 7 days or are accompanied by a fever, consult a doctor. Do not take this product if you have heart disease, high blood pressure, diabetes, thyroid disease, or difficulty in urination due to enlargement of the prostate gland unless directed by a doctor. Do not give this product to a child who has heart disease, high blood pressure, diabetes or thyroid disease. DRUG INTERACTION PRECAUTION: Do not use this product if you are now taking a prescription drug for high blood pressure without first consulting your doctor or if you are now taking a prescription monoamine oxidase inhibitor (MAOI) (certain drugs for depression, psychiatric or emotional conditions, or Parkinson's disease) or for 2 weeks after stopping the MAOI drug. If you are uncertain if your prescription drug contains an MAOI, consult a health professional before taking this product.

CITRUCEL FIBER THERAPY FOR REGULARITY
SmithKline Beecham
Consumer Health Care, L.P.

Dosage Form: powder

Active Ingredient: methylcellulose

Warning: Do not use laxative products when abdominal pain, nausea, or vomiting are present unless directed by a doctor. If you have noticed a sudden change in bowel habits that persists over a period of 2 weeks, consult a doctor before using a laxative. Laxative products should not be used for a period longer than 1 week unless directed by a doctor. Discontinue use and consult a doctor if rectal bleeding or failure to have a bowel movement occurs after using any laxative product. Unless recommended by a doctor do not exceed recommended maximum daily dose. If sensitive to any of the ingredients do not use. TAKING THIS PRODUCT WITHOUT ADEQUATE FLUID MAY CAUSE IT TO SWELL AND BLOCK YOUR THROAT OR ESOPHAGUS AND MAY CAUSE CHOKING. DO NOT TAKE THIS PRODUCT IF YOU HAVE DIFFICULTY IN SWALLOWING. IF YOU EXPERIENCE CHEST PAIN, VOMITING, OR DIFFICULTY IN SWALLOWING OR BREATHING AFTER TAKING THIS PRODUCT SEEK IMMEDIATE MEDICAL ATTENTION.

CLEAN & CLEAR DEEP ACTION CREAM CLEANSER
Johnson & Johnson
Consumer Products, Inc.

Dosage Form: cream

Active Ingredient: salicylic acid

Warning: For external use only. Avoid contact with the eyes. If contact occurs, flush thoroughly with water.

CLEAN & CLEAR INVISIBLE BLEMISH TREATMENT
Johnson & Johnson
Consumer Products, Inc.

Dosage Form: gel

Active Ingredient: salicylic acid

Warning: For external use only. Avoid contact with eyes. If contact occurs, flush thoroughly with water. Using other topical acne medications at the same time or immediately following use of this product may increase dryness or irritation of the skin. If this occurs, only one medication should be used unless directed by a doctor.

CLEAN & CLEAR PERSA-GEL EXTRA STRENGTH
Johnson & Johnson
Consumer Products, Inc.

Dosage Form: gel

Active Ingredient: benzoyl peroxide

Warning: When using any product containing benzoyl peroxide avoid any unnecessary sun exposure and use a sunscreen. For external use only. Keep away from eyes, lips, mouth and sensitive areas of the neck. If contact with eyes occurs, flush thoroughly with water. Using other topical acne medications at the same time or immediately following use of this product may increase dryness or irritation of the skin. If this occurs, only one medication should be used unless directed by a doctor. Do not use this medication if you have very sensitive skin or are sensitive to benzoyl peroxide. This product may cause irritation, characterized by redness, burning, itching, peeling, or possibly swelling. More frequent use or higher concentrations may aggravate such irritation. Mild irritation may be reduced by using the product less frequently or in a lower concentration. If irritation becomes severe, discontinue use; if irritation still continues consult your doctor. This product may bleach hair or dyed fabrics.

CLEAR EYES LUBRICANT EYE REDNESS RELIEVER
Ross Products/Abbott Laboratories

Dosage Form: drops

Active Ingredients: glycerin, naphazoline hydrochloride (HCl)

Warning: To avoid contamination do not touch tip of container to any surface. Replace cap after usage. If you experience eye pain, changes in vision, continued redness or irritation of the eye, or if the condition worsens or persists for more than 72 hours, discontinue use and consult a doctor. If you have glaucoma, do not use this product except under the advice and supervision of a doctor. Overuse of this product may produce increased redness of the eye. If the solution changes color or becomes cloudy, do not use.

CLEAR TOTAL LICE TREATMENT ELIMINATION SYSTEM LICE KILLING SHAMPOO AND LICE EGG REMOVER
Care Technologies, Inc.

Dosage Form: *Shampoo:* liquid
Lice Egg Remover: gel

Active Ingredients:
Shampoo: pyrethrum extract, piperonyl butoxide

Lice Egg Remover: No active ingredients have been indicated by the manufacturer.

Warning: *Shampoo:*Use with caution on persons allergic to ragweed. For external use only. Do not use near the eyes or permit contact with mucous membranes such as inside the nose, mouth, or vagina, as irritation may occur. Keep out of eyes when rinsing hair. *Adults and children:* Close eyes tightly and do not open eyes until product is rinsed out. Also, protect children's eyes with washcloth, towel or other suitable material, or by similar method. If product gets into the eyes, immediately flush with water. If

skin irritation or infection is present or develops, discontinue use and consult a doctor. Consult a doctor if infestation of eyebrows or eyelashes occurs.

CLEARASIL ANTIBACTERIAL SOAP
The Procter & Gamble Company

Dosage Form: cleansing bar

Active Ingredient: triclosan

Warning: Do not use this product on children under 6 months of age.

CLEARASIL CLEARSTICK MAXIMUM STRENGTH
The Procter & Gamble Company

Dosage Form: liquid

Active Ingredient: salicylic acid

Warning: For external use only. Avoid contact with eyes. If contact occurs, flush thoroughly with water. Using other topical acne medications at the same time or immediately following use of this product may increase dryness or irritation of the skin. If this occurs, only one medication should be used unless directed by a doctor.

CLEARASIL DAILY FACE WASH
The Procter & Gamble Company

Dosage Form: lotion

Active Ingredient: triclosan

Warning: Do not use this product on children under 6 months of age.

CLEARASIL MAXIMUM STRENGTH VANISHING OR TINTED CREAM
The Procter & Gamble Company

Dosage Form: cream

Active Ingredient: benzoyl peroxide

Warning: For external use only. Keep away from eyes, lips, mouth and sensitive areas of the neck. If contact with eyes occurs, flush thoroughly with water. Using other topical acne medications at the same time or immediately following use of this product may increase dryness or irritation of the skin. If this occurs only one medication should be used unless directed by a doctor. Do not use this medication if you have very sensitive skin or if you are sensitive to benzoyl peroxide. This product may cause irritation, characterized by redness, burning, itching, peeling or possibly swelling. More frequent use or higher concentrations may aggravate such irritation. Mild irritation may be reduced by using the product less frequently or in a lower concentration. If irritation becomes severe, discontinue use; if irritation still continues consult a doctor. This product may bleach hair or dyed fabrics.

CLEARASIL ULTRA PADS WITH ALOE
The Procter & Gamble Company

Dosage Form: pad

Active Ingredient: salicylic acid

Warning: For external use only. Avoid contact with eyes. If contact occurs, flush thoroughly with water. Using other topical acne medications at the same time or immediately following use of this product may increase dryness or irritation of the skin. If this occurs, only one acne medication should be used unless directed by a doctor.

COLA SYRUP
Unico Holding Company

Dosage Form: syrup

Active Ingredient: No active ingredients have been indicated by the manufacturer.

Warning: This product contains fructose and should not be taken by persons with hereditary fructose intolerence (HFI). This product contains sugar and should not be taken by diabetics except under the advice and supervision of a doctor. If nausea continues or recurs frequently consult a doctor.

COLACE
Roberts Pharmaceutical Corporation

Dosage Form: capsule, liquid, syrup

Active Ingredient: docusate sodium

Warning: Do not use this product when abdominal pain, nausea or vomiting are present, unless directed by a doctor. If you have noticed a sudden change in bowel habits that persists over a period of 2 weeks, consult a doctor before using a laxative. Laxative products should not be used for a period longer than 1 week unless directed by a doctor. Rectal bleeding or failure to have a bowel movement after use of a laxative may indicate a serious condition. Discontinue use and consult a doctor.

COMPOUND W WART REMOVER
Whitehall-Robins Healthcare

Dosage Form: gel, liquid

Active Ingredient: salicylic acid

Warning: For external use only. Do not use this product on irritated skin, on any area that is infected or reddened, if you are a diabetic, or if you have poor blood circulation. Serious complications may result. If discomfort persists, see your doctor. Do not use on moles, birthmarks, warts with hair growing from them, genital warts, warts on the face or mucous membranes (inside mouth, nose, anus, genitals or on lips). If product gets in the eyes, flush with water for 15 minutes. Extremely flammable. Keep away from fire or flame. Avoid smoking during application and until product has dried. Cap bottle tightly and store at room temperature away from heat. Avoid inhaling vapors.

COMPOZ NIGHTTIME SLEEP AID MAXIMUM STRENGTH
Medtech Laboratories, Inc.

Dosage Form: caplet

Active Ingredient: diphenhydramine hydrochloride (HCl)

Warning: Do not give to children under 12 years of age. If sleeplessness persists continuously for more than 2 weeks, consult a doctor. Insomnia may be a symptom of serious underlying medical illness. Do not take this product unless directed by a doctor, if you have breathing problems such as emphysema or chronic bronchitis, or if you have glaucoma, or difficulty in urination due to enlargement of the prostate gland. Avoid alcoholic beverages while taking this product. Do not take this product if you are taking sedatives or tranquilizers without first consulting your doctor.

COMTREX MAXIMUM STRENGTH ALLERGY-SINUS TREATMENT
Bristol-Myers Products

Dosage Form: caplet, tablet

Active Ingredient: pseudoephedrine hydrochloride (HCl), chlorpheniramine maleate, acetaminophen

Warning: Do not exceed recommended dosage because at higher dosages, nervousness, dizziness, or sleeplessness may occur. Do not take this product for pain or congestion for more than 7 days and do not take for fever for more than 3 days unless directed by a doctor. If pain or fever persists or gets worse, if new symptoms occur or if redness or swelling is persistent, consult a doctor because these could be signs of a serious condition. Do not take this product if you have a breathing problem such as emphysema or chronic bronchitis, or if you have heart disease, high blood pressure, diabetes, thyroid disease, glaucoma, or difficulty in urination due to enlargement of the prostate gland unless directed by a doctor. May cause excitability especially in children. May cause drowsiness; alcohol, sedatives, and tranquilizers may increase its drowsiness effect. Avoid alcoholic beverages while taking this product. Do not take this product if you are taking sedatives or tranquilizers without first consulting your doctor. Use caution while driving a motor vehicle or operating machinery. Do not use with other products containing acetaminophen. DRUG INTERACTION PRECAUTION: Do not use this product if you are now taking a prescription drug for high blood pressure without first consulting your doctor or if you are now taking a prescription monoamine oxidase inhibitor (MAOI) (certain drugs for depression, psychiatric or emotional conditions, or Parkinson's disease) or for 2 weeks after stopping the MAOI drug. If you are uncertain if your prescription drug contains an MAOI, consult a health professional before taking this product.

COMTREX MAXIMUM STRENGTH MULTI-SYMPTOM COLD & FLU RELIEF
Bristol-Myers Products

Dosage Form: caplet, tablet, liquid

Active Ingredient: pseudoephedrine hydrochloride (HCl), chlorpheniramine maleate, acetaminophen, dextromethorphan hydrobromide

Warning: Do not exceed recommended dosage. If nervousness, dizziness, or sleeplessness occur, discontinue use and consult a doctor. Do not take this product for more than 7 days. If symptoms do not improve within 7 days or are accompanied by a fever that lasts for more than 3 days, or if new symptoms occur, or if redness or swelling is present, consult a doctor. If cough persists for more than 1 week, tends to recur, or is accompanied by a rash, persistent headache, a fever that lasts for more than 3 days, or if new symptoms occur, consult a doctor. A persistent cough may be a sign of a serious condition. Do not take this product for persistent or chronic cough such as occurs with smoking, asthma, emphysema, or if cough is accompanied by excessive phlegm (mucous) unless directed by a doctor. Do not take this product, if you have a breathing problem such as emphysema or chronic bronchitis, or if you have glaucoma, high blood pressure, heart disease, thyroid disease, diabetes or difficulty in urination due to the enlargement of the prostate gland, without first consulting a doctor. May cause excitability especially in children. May cause marked drowsiness; alcohol, sedatives, and tranquilizers may increase its drowsiness effect. Avoid alcoholic beverages while taking this product. Do not take this product if you are taking sedatives or tranquilizers without first consulting your doctor. Use caution while driving a motor vehicle or operating machinery. Do not use with other products containing acetaminophen. DRUG INTERACTION PRECAUTION: Do not use this product if you are now taking a prescription monoamine oxidase inhibitor (MAOI) (certain drugs for depression, psychiatric or emotional conditions, or Parkinson's disease) or for 2 weeks after stopping the MAOI drug. If you are uncertain if your prescription drug contains an MAOI, consult a health professional before taking this product.

CONTAC 12 HOUR COLD
SmithKline Beecham
Consumer Health Care, L.P.

Dosage Form: timed-release capsule

Active Ingredients: phenylpropanolamine hydrochloride (HCl), chlorpheniramine maleate

Warning: Do not exceed recommended dosage because at higher dosages, nervousness, dizziness, or sleeplessness may occur. If symptoms do not improve within 7 days or are accompanied by a fever, consult a doctor. Do not take this product if you have a breathing problem such as emphysema or chronic bronchitis, or if you have heart disease, high blood pressure, diabetes, thyroid disease, glaucoma or difficulty in urination due to enlargement of the prostate gland unless directed by a doctor. May cause excitability especially in children. May cause drowsiness; alcohol, sedatives, and tranquilizers may increase its drowsiness effect. Avoid alcoholic beverages while taking this product. Do not take this product if you are taking sedatives or tranquilizers without first consulting your doctor. Use caution while driving a motor vehicle or operating machinery. Do not chew or crush tablets. Swallow whole. Do not take this product if you are taking another medication containing phenylpropanolamine. DRUG INTERACTION PRECAUTION: Do not use this product if you are now taking a prescription monoamine oxidase inhibitor (MAOI) (certain drugs for depression, psychiatric or emotional conditions, or Parkinson's disease) or for 2 weeks after stopping the MAOI drug. If you are uncertain if your prescription drug contains an MAOI, consult a health professional before taking this product.

CONTAC SEVERE COLD & FLU MAXIMUM STRENGTH
SmithKline Beecham
Consumer Health Care, L.P.

Dosage Form: liquid

Active Ingredients: phenylpropanolamine hydrochloride (HCl), chlorpheniramine maleate, acetaminophen, dextromethorphan hydrobromide

Warning: Do not exceed recommended dosage. If nervousness, dizziness, or sleeplessness occur, discontinue use and consult a doctor. Do not take this product for more than 10 days. If symptoms do not improve or are accompanied by a fever that lasts for more than 3 days, or if new symptoms occur, or if redness or swelling is present, consult a doctor. If sore throat is severe, persists for more than 2 days, or is accompanied or followed by a fever, headache, rash, nausea or vomiting, consult a doctor promptly. If cough persists for more than 1 week, tends to recur, or is accompanied by a rash, persistent headache, a fever that lasts for more than 3 days, or if new symptoms occur, consult a doctor. A persistent cough may be a sign of a serious condition. Do not take this product for persistent or chronic cough such as occurs with smoking, asthma, emphysema, or if cough is accompanied by excessive phlegm (mucous) unless directed by a doctor. Do not take this product, if you have a breathing problem such as emphysema or chronic bronchitis, if you have glaucoma, high blood pressure, heart disease, thyroid disease, diabetes or difficulty in urination due to the enlargement of the prostate gland, without first consulting a doctor. May cause excitability especially in children. May cause marked drowsiness; alcohol, sedatives, and tranquilizers may increase its drowsiness effect. Avoid alcoholic beverages while taking this product. Do not take this product if you are taking sedatives or tranquilizers without first consulting your doctor. Use caution while driving a motor vehicle or operating machinery. DRUG INTERACTION PRECAUTION: Do not use this product if you are now taking a prescription monoamine oxidase inhibitor (MAOI) (certain drugs for depression, psychiatric or emotional conditions, or Parkinson's disease) or for 2 weeks after stopping the MAOI drug. If you are uncertain if your prescription drug contains an MAOI, consult a health professional before taking this product. Do not take this product if you are taking an appetite-controlling medication containing phenylpropanolamine. Do not use with other products containing acetaminophen.

CORICIDIN 'D'
Schering-Plough HealthCare Products

Dosage Form: tablet

Active Ingredients: phenylpropanolamine hydrochloride (HCl), chlorpheniramine maleate, acetaminophen

Warning: Do not exceed recommended dosage because at higher dosages, nervousness, dizziness, or sleeplessness may occur. If congestion does not improve within 7 days, consult a doctor. Do not take for pain for more than 10 days (adults) or 5 days (children 6 to under 12 years) or for fever for more than 3 days unless directed by a doctor. If pain or fever persists or gets worse, if new symptoms occur, or if redness or swelling is present, consult a doctor because these could be signs of serious illness. Do not take this product if you have a breathing

problem such as emphysema or chronic bronchitis, or if you have heart disease, high blood pressure, diabetes, thyroid disease, glaucoma, or difficulty in urination due to enlargement of the prostate gland unless directed by a doctor. May cause excitability especially in children. May cause drowsiness: alcohol, sedatives, and tranquilizers may increase its drowsiness effect. Avoid alcoholic beverages while taking this product. Do not take this product if you are taking sedatives or tranquilizers without first consulting your doctor. Use caution while driving a motor vehicle or operating machinery. Do not use with other products containing acetaminophen. DRUG INTERACTION PRECAUTION: Do not use this product if you are now taking a prescription monoamine oxidase inhibitor (MAOI) (certain drugs for depression, psychiatric or emotional conditions, or Parkinson's disease) or for 2 weeks after stopping the MAOI drug. If you are uncertain if your prescription drug contains an MAOI, consult a health professional before taking this product. Do not take this product if you are taking an appetite-controlling medication containing phenylpropanolamine.

CORRECTOL BISACODYL STIMULANT LAXATIVE
Schering-Plough HealthCare Products

Dosage Form: caplet, tablet

Active Ingredient: bisacodyl

Warning: Do not chew tablets or capsules. Do not give to children under 6 years of age, or to persons who can not swallow without chewing, unless directed by a doctor. Do not take this product within 1 hour after taking an antacid or milk. Do not use laxative products when abdominal pain, nausea, or vomiting are present unless directed by a doctor. If you have noticed a sudden change in bowel habits that persists over a period of 2 weeks, consult a doctor before using a laxative. Laxative products should not be used for a period longer than 1 week unless directed by a doctor. Rectal bleeding or failure to have a bowel movement after use of a laxative may indicate a serious condition. Discontinue use and consult a doctor. This product may cause abdominal discomfort, faintness and cramps.

CORTAID MAXIMUM STRENGTH
Pharmacia & Upjohn, Inc.

Dosage Form: ointment, cream

Active Ingredient: hydrocortisone

Warning: For external use only. Avoid contact with the eyes. If condition worsens, or if symptoms persist for more than 7 days or clear up and occur again within a few days, stop use of this product and do not begin use of any other hydrocortisone product unless you have consulted a doctor. Do not use for the treatment of diaper rash. Consult a doctor. For external feminine itching, do not use if you have a vaginal discharge. Consult a doctor. WARNING FOR EXTERNAL ANAL ITCHING USERS: Do not exceed the recommended daily dosage unless directed by a doctor. In case of bleeding, consult a doctor promptly. Do not put this product into the rectum by using fingers or any mechanical device or applicator.

CORTICAINE MAXIMUM STRENGTH
UCB Pharma, Inc.

Dosage Form: cream

Active Ingredient: hydrocortisone

Warning: For external use only. Avoid contact with the eyes. If condition worsens, or if symptoms persist for more than 7 days or clear up and occur again within a few days, stop use of this product and do not begin use of any other hydrocortisone product unless you have consulted a doctor. Do not use for the treatment of diaper rash. Consult a doctor. WARNING FOR EXTERNAL ANAL ITCHING USERS: Do not exceed the recommended daily dosage unless directed by a doctor. In case of bleeding, consult a doctor promptly. Do not put this product into the rectum by using fingers or any mechanical device or applicator.

CORTIZONE-10
Thompson Medical Company, Inc.

Dosage Form: cream, ointment

Active Ingredient: hydrocortisone

Warning: For external use only. Avoid contact with the eyes. If condition worsens, or if symptoms persist for more than 7 days or clear up and occur again within a few days, stop use of this product and do not begin use of any other hydrocortisone product unless you have consulted a doctor. Do not use for the treatment of diaper rash. Consult a doctor. Do not use in genital areas if you have a vaginal discharge. Consult a doctor. WARNING FOR EXTERNAL ANAL ITCHING USERS: Do not exceed the recommended daily dosage unless directed by a doctor. In case of bleeding, consult a doctor promptly. Do not put this product into the rectum by using fingers or any mechanical device or applicator.

COUGH-X
B. F. Ascher & Company, Inc.

Dosage Form: lozenge

Active Ingredient: benzocaine, dextromethorphan hydrobromide

Warning: A persistent cough may be a sign of a serious condition. If cough persists for more than 1 week, tends to recur, or is accompanied by a fever, rash or persistent headache, consult a doctor. Do not take this product for persistent or chronic cough such as occurs with smoking, asthma, emphysema, or if cough is accompanied by excessive phlegm (mucous) unless directed by a doctor. DRUG INTERACTION PRECAUTION: Do not use this product if you are now taking a prescription monoamine oxidase inhibitor (MAOI) (certain drugs for depression, psychiatric or emotional conditions, or Parkinson's disease) or for 2 weeks after stopping the MAOI drug. If you are uncertain if your prescription drug contains an MAOI, consult a health professional before taking this product.

CRUEX ANTIFUNGAL
Ciba Self-Medication, Inc. *

Dosage Form: spray powder, cream

Active Ingredient: undecylenate (as undecylenic acid and zinc undecylenate)

Warning: For external use only. Do not use on children under 2 years of age unless directed by a doctor. Avoid contact with the eyes. If irritation occurs, or if there is no improvement within 4 weeks (for athlete's foot or ringworm) or within 2 weeks (for jock itch), discontinue use and consult a doctor or pharmacist. *For spray powder only:* Avoid inhaling. Avoid contact with the eyes and other mucous membranes. Contents under pressure. Do not puncture or incinerate. Flammable mixture, do not use while smoking or near fire or flame. Do not expose to heat or temperatures above 49°C (120°F.). Use only as directed. Intentional misuse by deliberately concentrating and inhaling the contents can be harmful or fatal.

CURÉL THERAPEUTIC MOISTURIZING
Bausch & Lomb
Personal Products Division

Dosage Form: lotion, cream

Active Ingredient: No active ingredients have been indicated by the manufacturer

Warning: For external use only.

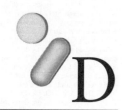

DEBROX DROPS
EARWAX REMOVAL AID
SmithKline Beecham
Consumer Health Care, L.P.

Dosage Form: drops

Active Ingredient: carbamide peroxide

Warning: Do not use if you have ear damage or discharge, ear pain, irritation or rash in the ear, or are dizzy; consult a doctor. Do not use if you have an injury or perforation (hole) of the eardrum or after ear surgery unless directed by a doctor. Avoid contact with the eyes. Do not use for more than 4 days. If excessive ear wax remains after use of this product, consult a doctor.

DELSYM 12 HOUR COUGH RELIEF
COUGH FORMULA
Fisons

Dosage Form: suspension

Active Ingredient: dextromethorphan polistirex

Warning: A persistent cough may be a sign of a serious condition. If cough persists for more than 1 week, tends to recur, or is accompanied by a fever, rash, or persistent headache consult a doctor. Do not take this product for persistent or chronic cough such as occurs with smoking, asthma, chronic bronchitis, emphysema, or if cough is accompanied by excessive phlegm (mucous) unless directed by a doctor. DRUG INTERACTION PRECAUTION: Do not use this product if you are now taking a prescription monoamine oxidase inhibitor (MAOI)

(certain drugs for depression, psychiatric or emotional conditions, or Parkinson's disease) or for 2 weeks after stopping the MAOI drug. If you are uncertain if your prescription drug contains an MAOI, consult a health professional before taking this product.

DENOREX MEDICATED SHAMPOO
Whitehall-Robins Healthcare

Dosage Form: shampoo

Active Ingredient: coal tar solution

Warning: For external use only. Avoid contact with the eyes. If contact occurs, rinse eyes thoroughly with water. If condition worsens or does not improve after regular use of this product as directed, consult a doctor. Use caution in exposing skin to sunlight after applying this product. It may increase tendency to sunburn for up to 24 hours after application. Do not use for prolonged periods without consulting a doctor. Do not use this product with other forms of psoriasis therapy, such as ultraviolet radiation or prescription drugs, unless directed by a doctor. If condition covers large area of the body, consult your doctor before using this product.

DENT'S MAXI-STRENGTH
TOOTHACHE TREATMENT
C. S. Dent & Company

Dosage Form: drops

Active Ingredient: benzocaine

Warning: Use as directed. Apply drops to tooth only. Avoid getting on gums. For temporary use only or until a dentist can be consulted. Do not use this product if you have a history of allergy to local anesthetics such as procaine, butacaine, benzocaine, or other "caine" anesthetics.

DERMAREST
Del Pharmaceuticals, Inc.

Dosage Form: gel

Active Ingredient: diphenhydramine hydrochloride (HCl)

Warning: For external use only. Avoid contact with the eyes. If condition worsens, does not improve within 7 days, or if symptoms persist for more than 7 days or clear up and occur again within a few days, discontinue use and consult a doctor. Do not use on chicken pox, measles, blisters or on extensive areas of skin, except as directed by a doctor. Do not use with any other drugs containing diphenhydramine while using this product.

DERMASIL DRY SKIN TREATMENT
Chesebrough-Pond's USA Company

Dosage Form: cream, lotion

Active Ingredient: dimethicone

Warning: For external use only. Avoid contact with eyes. If condition worsens or does not improve within 7 days, consult a doctor or pharmacist. Not to be applied over deep or puncture wounds, infections, or lacerations.

DERMOPLAST
Medtech

Dosage Form: spray, lotion

Active Ingredients: benzocaine, menthol

Warning: For external use only. Avoid contact with the eyes. If condition worsens, if a rash or irritation devel-

ops, or if symptoms persist for more than 7 days or clear up and occur again within a few days, discontinue use of this product and consult a doctor. Certain persons can develop allergic reactions to ingredients in this product. Do not use this product if you have a history of allergy to local anesthetics such as procaine, butacaine, benzocaine, or other "caine" anesthetics. Do not use in the eyes or apply over large areas of the body. Contents under pressure. Do not puncture or incinerate or expose to heat or temperature above 120°F . Flammable mixture; do not use near fire or throw into fire. Use only as directed. Intentional misuse by deliberately concentrating and inhaling the contents can be harmful or fatal.

DESENEX ANTIFUNGAL
*Ciba Self-Medication, Inc.**

Dosage Form: cream, ointment, powder, aerosol spray powder

Active Ingredient: undecylenate (as undecylenic acid and zinc undecylenate)

Warning: For external use only. Do not use on children under 2 years of age unless directed by a doctor. Avoid contact with the eyes. If irritation occurs, or if there is no improvement within 4 weeks (for athlete's foot or ringworm) or within 2 weeks (for jock itch), discontinue use and consult a doctor or pharmacist. *For spray powder only:* Avoid inhaling. Avoid contact with the eyes and other mucous membranes. Contents under pressure. Do not puncture or incinerate. Flammable mixture, do not use while smoking or near fire or flame. Do not expose to heat or temperatures above 49°C (120°F). Use only as directed. Intentional misuse by deliberately concentrating and inhaling the contents can be harmful or fatal.

DESENEX PRESCRIPTION STRENGTH
*Ciba Self-Medication, Inc.**

Dosage Form: cream

Active Ingredient: clotrimazole

Warning: For external use only. Do not use on children under 2 years of age unless directed by a doctor. Avoid contact with the eyes. If irritation occurs or if there is no improvement within 4 weeks (for athlete's foot or ringworm) or within 2 weeks (for jock itch), discontinue use and consult a doctor or pharmacist.

Dosage Form: liquid spray, spray powder

Active Ingredient: miconazole nitrate

Warning: For external use only. Do not use on children under 2 years of age unless directed by a doctor. If irritation occurs or if there is no improvement within 4 weeks (for athlete's foot or ringworm) or within 2 weeks (for jock itch), discontinue use and consult a doctor or pharmacist. Avoid inhaling. Avoid contact with the eyes and other mucous membranes. Contents under pressure. Do not puncture or incinerate. Flammable mixture, do not use while smoking or near fire or flame. Do not expose to heat or temperatures above 49°C (120°F). Use only as directed. Intentional misuse by deliberately concentrating and inhaling the contents can be harmful or fatal.

DESITIN CORNSTARCH BABY POWDER
Pfizer Inc., Consumer Care Group

Dosage Form: powder

Active Ingredients: corn starch, zinc oxide

Warning: For external use only. Do not use on broken skin. Avoid contact with eyes. Keep powder away from child's face to avoid inhalation. If diaper rash worsens or does not improve within 7 days consult your doctor.

DESITIN DIAPER RASH OINTMENT
Pfizer Inc., Consumer Care Group

Dosage Form: ointment

Active Ingredients: zinc oxide

Warning: No other warnings other than those listed at the beginning of this section have been indicated by the manufacturer.

DI-GEL ANTACID/ANTI-GAS
Schering-Plough HealthCare Products

Dosage Form: liquid

Active Ingredient: simethicone, aluminum hydroxide, magnesium hydroxide

Dosage Form: chewable tablet

Active Ingredient: simethicone, magnesium hydroxide

Warning: Do not exceed recommended daily dosage, or use the maximum dosage of this product for more than 2 weeks. Do not use this product if you have kidney disease, except under the advice and supervision of a doctor. DRUG INTERACTION PRECAUTION: Antacids may interact with certain prescription drugs. Do not use take this product if you are presently taking a prescription antibiotic drug containing any form of tetracycline.

DIAPARENE CORNSTARCH BABY POWDER
*Personal Care Group, Inc.
c/o Reckitt & Colman*

Dosage Form: powder

Active Ingredient: corn starch

Warning: For external use only. Avoid contact with eyes. If condition worsens or does not improve within 7 days, consult a doctor. Do not use on broken skin. Keep powder away from child's face to avoid inhalation, which can cause breathing problems.

DIAPARENE DIAPER RASH OINTMENT
*Personal Care Group, Inc.
c/o Reckitt & Colman*

Dosage Form: ointment

Active Ingredient: zinc oxide

Warning: For external use only. Avoid contact with eyes. If condition worsens or does not improve within 7 days, consult a doctor. Not to be applied over puncture wounds, infections or lacerations.

DIMETAPP 4-HOUR MAXIMUM STRENGTH
Whitehall-Robins Healthcare

Dosage Form: tablet, softgel

Active Ingredients: phenylpropanolamine hydrochloride (HCl), brompheniramine maleate

Warning: Do not exceed recommended dosage because at higher dosages, nervousness, dizziness, or sleeplessness

may occur. If symptoms do not improve within 7 days or are accompanied by a fever, consult a doctor. Do not take this product if you have a breathing problem such as emphysema or chronic bronchitis, or if you have heart disease, high blood pressure, diabetes, thyroid disease, glaucoma or difficulty in urination due to enlargement of the prostate gland, unless directed by a doctor. May cause excitability especially in children. May cause drowsiness; alcohol, sedatives, and tranquilizers may increase its drowsiness effect. Avoid alcoholic beverages while taking this product. Do not take this product if you are taking sedatives or tranquilizers without first consulting your doctor. Use caution while driving a motor vehicle or operating machinery. Do not take this product if you are taking another medication containing phenylpropanolamine. DRUG INTERACTION PRECAUTION: Do not use this product if you are now taking a prescription monoamine oxidase inhibitor (MAOI) (certain drugs for depression, psychiatric or emotional conditions, or Parkinson's disease) or for 2 weeks after stopping the MAOI drug. If you are uncertain if your prescription drug contains an MAOI, consult a health professional before taking this product.

DIMETAPP ALLERGY
Whitehall-Robins Healthcare

Dosage Form: tablet, softgel

Active Ingredient: brompheniramine maleate

Warning: May cause excitability especially in children. Do not take this product if you have asthma, glaucoma, emphysema, chronic pulmonary disease, shortness of breath, difficulty in breathing, or difficulty in urination due to enlargement of the prostate gland unless directed by a doctor. May cause drowsiness; alcohol, sedatives, and tranquilizers may increase its drowsiness effect. Avoid alcoholic beverages while taking this product. Do not take this product if you are taking sedatives or tranquilizers without first consulting your doctor. Use caution while driving a motor vehicle or operating machinery. Do not take this product if you are hypersensitive to any of the ingredients.

DIMETAPP ALLERGY DYE-FREE ELIXIR
Whitehall-Robins Healthcare

Dosage Form: elixir

Active Ingredient: brompheniramine maleate

Warning: May cause excitability especially in children. Do not take this product if you have breathing problems such as emphysema or chronic bronchitis, or if you have glaucoma, or difficulty in urination due to enlargement of the prostate gland unless directed by a doctor. May cause drowsiness; alcohol, sedatives, and tranquilizers may increase its drowsiness effect. Avoid alcoholic beverages while taking this product. Do not take this product while taking sedatives or tranquilizers without first consulting your doctor. Use caution while driving a motor vehicle or operating machinery.

DIMETAPP ALLERGY SINUS
Whitehall-Robins Healthcare

Dosage Form: caplet

Active Ingredients: phenylpropanolamine hydrochloride (HCl), brompheniramine maleate, acetaminophen

Warning: Do not exceed recommended dosage because at higher dosages, nervousness, dizziness, or sleeplessness may occur. Do not take for pain for more than 7 days or for fever for more than 3 days unless directed by a doctor. If pain or fever persists, or gets worse, if new symptoms occur, or if redness or swelling is present, consult a doctor because these could be signs of a serious condition. Do not take this product if you have a breathing problem such as emphysema or chronic bronchitis, or if you have heart disease, high blood pressure, diabetes, thyroid disease, glaucoma or difficulty in urination due to enlargement of the prostate gland unless directed by a doctor. May cause excitability especially in children. May cause drowsiness; alcohol, sedatives, and tranquilizers may increase its drowsiness effect. Avoid alcoholic beverages while taking this product. Do not take this product while taking sedatives or tranquilizers without first consulting your doctor. If you generally consume 3 or more alcohol-containing drinks per day, you should consult your doctor for advice on when and how you should take this product or any other acetaminophen-containing product. Use caution while driving a motor vehicle or operating machinery. DRUG INTERACTION PRECAUTION: Do not use this product if you are now taking a prescription monoamine oxidase inhibitor (MAOI) (certain drugs for depression, psychiatric or emotional conditions, or Parkinson's disease) or for 2 weeks after stopping the MAOI drug. If you are uncertain if your prescription drug contains an MAOI, consult a health professional before taking this product. Do not take this product if you are taking another medication containing phenylpropanolamine.

DIMETAPP COLD & ALLERGY
Whitehall-Robins Healthcare

Dosage Form: chewable tablet, quick dissolve tablet

Active Ingredients: phenylpropanolamine hydrochloride (HCl), brompheniramine maleate

Warning: Do not exceed recommended dosage because at higher dosages, nervousness, dizziness, or sleeplessness may occur. If symptoms do not improve within 7 days or are accompanied by a fever, consult a doctor. Do not take this product if you have a breathing problem such as emphysema or chronic bronchitis, heart disease, high blood pressure, diabetes, thyroid disease, or if you have glaucoma or difficulty in urination due to enlargement of the prostate gland unless directed by a doctor. May cause excitability especially in children. May cause drowsiness; sedatives, and tranquilizers may increase its drowsiness effect. Do not give to children who are taking sedatives or tranquilizers without first consulting your doctor. Do not take this product if you are taking another medication containing phenyl-propanolamine. DRUG INTERAC-TION PRECAUTION: Do not use this product if you are now taking a prescription monoamine oxidase inhibitor (MAOI) (certain drugs for depression, psychiatric or emotional conditions, or Parkinson's disease) or for 2 weeks after stopping the MAOI drug. If you are uncertain if your prescription drug contains an MAOI, consult a health professional before taking this product. Do not use if you are presently taking another medication containing phenylpropanolamine, unless directed by a doctor.

DIMETAPP DECONGESTANT NON-DROWSY LIQUI-GELS
Whitehall-Robins Healthcare

Dosage Form: softgel

Active Ingredient: pseudoephedrine hydrochloride (HCl)

Warning: Do not exceed recommended dosage because at higher dosages, nervousness, dizziness, or sleeplessness may occur. If symptoms do not improve within 7 days or are accompanied by a fever, consult a doctor. Do not take this product if you have heart disease, high blood pressure, diabetes, thyroid disease, or difficulty in urination due to enlargement of the prostate gland unless directed by a doctor. DRUG INTERACTION PRECAUTION: Do not use this product if you are now taking a prescription monoamine oxidase inhibitor (MAOI) (certain drugs for depression, psychiatric or emotional conditions, or Parkinson's disease) or for 2 weeks after stopping the MAOI drug. If you are uncertain if your prescription drug contains an MAOI, consult a health professional before taking this product.

DIMETAPP DECONGESTANT PEDIATRIC DROPS
Whitehall-Robins Healthcare

Dosage Form: drops

Active Ingredient: pseudoephedrine hydrochloride (HCl)

Warning: Do not exceed recommended dosage because at higher dosages, nervousness, dizziness, or sleeplessness may occur. If symptoms do not improve within 7 days or are accompanied by a fever, consult a doctor. Do not give this product to a child who has heart disease, high blood pressure, thyroid disease, or diabetes unless directed by a doctor. DRUG INTERACTION PRECAUTION: Do not use this product if you are now taking a prescription monoamine oxidase inhibitor (MAOI) (certain drugs for depression, psychiatric or emotional conditions, or Parkinson's disease) or for 2 weeks after stopping the MAOI drug. If you are uncertain if your prescription drug contains an MAOI, consult a health professional before taking this product.

DOAN'S EXTRA STRENGTH
Ciba Self-Medication, Inc.*

Dosage Form: caplets

Active Ingredient: magnesium salicylate tetrahydrate

Warning: Children and teenagers should not use this medicine for chicken pox or flu symptoms before a doctor is consulted about Reye Syndrome,

a rare but serious illness. Do not take this product for pain for more than 10 days unless directed by a doctor. If pain or fever persists or gets worse, if new symptoms occur, or if redness or swelling is present, consult a doctor. These could be signs of serious illness. Do not take this product if you are allergic to salicylates (including aspirin), have stomach problems (such as heartburn, upset stomach or stomach pain) that persist or recur, or if you have ulcers or bleeding problems, unless directed by a doctor. If ringing in the ears or loss of hearing occurs, consult a doctor before taking any more of this product. DRUG INTERACTION PRECAUTION: Do not use if taking a prescription drug for anti-coagulation (blood thinning), diabetes, gout or arthritis unless directed by a doctor. IT IS ESPECIALLY IMPORTANT NOT TO USE ASPIRIN DURING THE LAST 3 MONTHS OF PREGNANCY UNLESS SPECIFICALLY DIRECTED TO DO SO BY A DOCTOR BECAUSE IT MAY CAUSE PROBLEMS IN THE UNBORN CHILD OR COMPLICATIONS DURING DELIVERY.

DONNAGEL
Wyeth-Ayerst Laboratories

Dosage Form: chewable tablet, suspension

Active Ingredient: attapulgite

Warning: Do not use for more than 2 days unless directed by a doctor. Do not use if diarrhea is accompanied by a fever, or if blood or mucus is present in the stool. Do not use in children under 6 years of age unless directed by a doctor. If you are taking a prescription medicine, consult your doctor before taking this product.

DORCOL CHILDREN'S COUGH SYRUP
Sandoz North American Consumer Pharmaceuticals

Dosage Form: syrup

Active Ingredients: pseudoephedrine hydrochloride (HCl), guaifenesin, dextromethorphan hydrobromide

Warning: Do not exceed recommended dosage because at higher dosages, nervousness, dizziness, or sleeplessness may occur. If symptoms do not improve within 7 days or are accompanied by a fever, consult a doctor. Do not give this product to a child who has heart disease, high blood pressure, thyroid disease, or diabetes unless directed by a doctor. A persistent cough may be a sign of a serious condition. If cough persists for more than 1 week, tends to recur, or is accompanied by a fever, rash or persistent headache, consult a doctor. Do not take this product for persistent or chronic cough such as occurs with asthma or if cough is accompanied by excessive phlegm (mucous) unless directed by a doctor. DRUG INTERACTION PRECAUTION: Do not use this product if you are now taking a prescription monoamine oxidase inhibitor (MAOI) (certain drugs for depression, psychiatric or emotional conditions, or Parkinson's disease) or for 2 weeks after stopping the MAOI drug. If you are uncertain if your prescription drug contains an MAOI, consult a health professional before taking this product.

DOXIDAN
Pharmacia & Upjohn, Inc.

Dosage Form: softgel

Active Ingredients: docusate sodium, casanthranol

Warning: Do not use laxative products when abdominal pain, nausea, or vomiting are present unless directed by a doctor. If you have noticed a sudden change in bowel habits that persists over a period of 2 weeks, consult a doctor before using a laxative. Laxative products should not be used for a period longer than 1 week unless directed by a doctor. Rectal bleeding or failure to have a bowel movement after use of a laxative may indicate a serious condition. Discontinue use and consult a doctor. If skin rash appears, do not use this product or any other preparation containing phenolphthalein. DRUG INTERACTION PRECAUTION: Do not take this product if you are presently taking mineral oil, unless directed by a doctor.

DR. SCHOLL'S ADVANCED PAIN RELIEF CALLUS REMOVERS
Schering-Plough HealthCare Products

Dosage Form: disc

Active Ingredient: salicylic acid

Warning: For external use only. Do not use this product on irritated skin, or any area that is infected or reddened, if you are a diabetic, or if you have poor blood circulation. If discomfort persists, see your doctor or podiatrist.

DR. SCHOLL'S ADVANCED PAIN RELIEF CORN REMOVERS
Schering-Plough HealthCare Products

Dosage Form: disc

Active Ingredient: salicylic acid

Warning: For external use only. Do not use this product on irritated skin, or any area that is infected or reddened, if you are a diabetic, or if you have poor blood circulation. If discomfort persists, see your doctor or podiatrist.

DR. SCHOLL'S ATHLETE'S FOOT
Schering-Plough HealthCare Products

Dosage Form: powder, spray liquid

Active Ingredient: tolnaftate

Warning: Do not use on children under 2 years of age unless directed by a doctor. For external use only. Avoid contact with the eyes. If irritation occurs or if there is no improvement within 4 weeks, discontinue use and consult a doctor.

DR. SCHOLL'S CLEAR AWAY ONE STEP SALICYLIC ACID WART REMOVER
Schering-Plough HealthCare Products

Dosage Form: disc, liquid

Active Ingredient: salicylic acid

Warning: For external use only. Do not use this product on irritated skin, on any area that is infected or reddened, if you are a diabetic, or if you have poor blood circulation. If discomfort persists, see your doctor. Do not use on moles, birthmarks, warts with hair growing from them, genital warts, warts on the face or mucous membranes.

DR. SCHOLL'S LIQUID CORN/CALLUS REMOVER
Schering-Plough HealthCare Products

Dosage Form: liquid

Active Ingredient: salicylic acid

Warning: For external use only. Do not apply more than 4 days. Do not use this product on irritated skin, or any area that is infected or reddened, if you are a diabetic, or if you have poor blood circulation. In these cases or when in doubt, use pad only and consult your doctor or podiatrist. Keep bottle tightly capped and away from flame.

DR. SCHOLL'S ONE STEP CALLUS REMOVERS
Schering-Plough HealthCare Products

Dosage Form: disc

Active Ingredient: salicylic acid

Warning: For external use only. Do not use this product on irritated skin, or any area that is infected or reddened, if you are a diabetic, or if you have poor blood circulation. If discomfort persists, see your doctor or podiatrist.

DR. SCHOLL'S ONE STEP CORN REMOVERS
Schering-Plough HealthCare Products

Dosage Form: strip

Active Ingredient: salicylic acid

Warning: For external use only. Do not use this product on irritated skin, or any area that is infected or reddened, if you are a diabetic, or if you have poor blood circulation. If discomfort persists, see your doctor or podiatrist.

DR. SCHOLL'S SOFT CORN REMOVERS
Schering-Plough HealthCare Products

Dosage Form: disc

Active Ingredient: salicylic acid

Warning: For external use only. Do not use this product on irritated skin, or any area that is infected or reddened, if you are a diabetic, or if you have poor blood circulation. If discomfort persists, see your doctor or podiatrist.

DR. SCHOLL'S WRAP-AROUND CORN REMOVERS
Schering-Plough HealthCare Products

Dosage Form: disc

Active Ingredient: salicylic acid

Warning: For external use only. Do not use this product on irritated skin, or any area that is infected or reddened, if you are a diabetic, or if you have poor blood circulation. If discomfort persists, see your doctor or podiatrist.

DRAMAMINE II LESS DROWSY FORMULA
Pharmacia & Upjohn, Inc.

Dosage Form: tablet

Active Ingredient: meclizine hydrochloride (HCl)

Warning: Do not give to children under 12 years of age unless directed by a doctor. Do not take this product, if you have breathing problems such as emphysema, or chronic bronchitis, or if you have glaucoma, or difficulty in urination due to enlargement of the prostate gland, unless directed by a doctor. May cause drowsiness; alco-

hol, sedatives, and tranquilizers may increase its drowsiness effect. Avoid alcoholic beverages while taking this product. Do not take this product if you are taking sedatives or tranquilizers without first consulting your doctor. Use caution when driving a motor vehicle or operating machinery. Not for frequent or prolonged use, except on advice of a doctor. Do not exceed recommended dosage.

DRAMAMINE ORIGINAL FORMULA
Pharmacia & Upjohn, Inc.

Dosage Form: tablet

Active Ingredient: dimenhydrinate

Warning: Do not give to children under 12 years of age unless directed by a doctor. Do not take this product if you have breathing problems such as emphysema, or chronic bronchitis, or if you have glaucoma, or difficulty in urination due to enlargement of the prostate gland, unless directed by a doctor. May cause drowsiness; alcohol, sedatives, and tranquilizers may increase its drowsiness effect. Avoid alcoholic beverages while taking this product. Do not take this product if you are taking sedatives or tranquilizers without first consulting your doctor. Use caution when driving a motor vehicle or operating machinery. Not for frequent or prolonged use, except on advice of a doctor. Do not exceed recommended dosage.

DRISTAN 12-HOUR NASAL SPRAY
Whitehall-Robins Healthcare

Dosage Form: spray

Active Ingredients: oxymetazoline hydrochloride (HCl)

Warning: Do not exceed recommended dosage. This product may cause temporary discomfort, such as burning, stinging, sneezing, or an increase in nasal discharge. Do not use for more than 3 days. Use only as directed. Frequent or prolonged use may cause nasal congestion to recur or worsen. If symptoms persist, consult a doctor. Do not take this product if you have heart disease, high blood pressure, thyroid disease, diabetes or difficulty in urination due to enlargement of the prostate gland unless directed by a doctor. Do not use this product on a child who has heart disease, high blood pressure, thyroid disease, or diabetes unless directed by a doctor. The use of this container by more than one person may spread infection.

DRISTAN COLD MULTI-SYMPTOM FORMULA
Whitehall-Robins Healthcare

Dosage Form: tablet

Active Ingredients: phenylephrine hydrochloride (HCl), chlorpheniramine maleate, acetaminophen

Warning: Do not exceed recommended dosage because at higher dosages, nervousness, dizziness, or sleeplessness may occur. Do not take this product for more than 7 days. If symptoms do not improve or are accompanied by fever that lasts for more than 3 days, if new symptoms occur, if redness or swelling is present, or if sore throat is severe, persists for more than 2 days, or is accompanied or followed by fever, headache, rash, nausea or vomiting, consult a doctor. Do not take

this product if you have a breathing problem such as emphysema or chronic bronchitis, or if you have heart disease, high blood pressure, diabetes, thyroid disease, glaucoma, or difficulty in urination due to enlargement of the prostate gland unless directed by a doctor. May cause excitability especially in children. May cause drowsiness; alcohol, sedatives, and tranquilizers may increase its drowsiness effect. Do not take this product if you are taking sedatives or tranquilizers without first consulting your doctor. Avoid alcoholic beverages while taking this product. If you generally consume 3 or more alcohol-containing drinks per day, you should consult your doctor for advice on when and how you should take this product or any other acetaminophen-containing product. Use caution while driving a motor vehicle or operating machinery. DRUG INTERACTION PRECAUTION: Do not use this product if you are now taking a prescription monoamine oxidase inhibitor (MAOI) (certain drugs for depression, psychiatric or emotional conditions, or Parkinson's disease) or for 2 weeks after stopping the MAOI drug. If you are uncertain if your prescription drug contains an MAOI, consult a health professional before taking this product.

DRISTAN SINUS
Whitehall-Robins Healthcare

Dosage Form: caplet

Active Ingredients: pseudoephedrine hydrochloride (HCl), ibuprofen

Warning: ASPIRIN SENSITIVE PATIENTS: Do not take this product if you have had a severe allergic reaction to aspirin, e.g.—asthma, swelling, shock or hives, because even though this product contains no aspirin or salicylates, cross-reactions may occur in patients allergic to aspirin. Do not exceed recommended dosage because at higher dosages, nervousness, dizziness, or sleeplessness may occur. Do not take for colds for more than 7 days or for fever for more than 3 days unless directed by a doctor. If the cold or fever persists or gets worse, or if new symptoms occur, consult a doctor. These could be signs of serious illness. If you are under a doctor's care for any serious condition, consult a doctor before taking this product. As with aspirin and acetaminophen, if you have any condition which requires you to take prescription drugs or if you have had any problems or serious side effects from taking any non-prescription pain reliever, do not take this product without first discussing it with your doctor. If you experience any symptoms which are unusual or seem unrelated to the condition for which you took this product, consult a doctor before taking any more of it. Do not take this product if you have heart disease, high blood pressure, thyroid disease, diabetes or difficulty in urination due to enlargement of the prostate gland, unless directed by a doctor. Do not combine this product with other non-prescription pain relievers. Do not combine this product with any other ibuprofen-containing product. DRUG INTERACTION PRECAUTION: Do not use this product if you are now taking a prescription monoamine oxidase inhibitor (MAOI) (certain drugs for depression, psychiatric or emotional conditions, or Parkinson's disease) or for 2 weeks after stopping the MAOI drug. If you are uncertain if your prescription drug contains an MAOI, consult a health professional before taking this product. IT IS ESPECIALLY IMPORTANT NOT TO USE ASPIRIN DURING THE LAST 3 MONTHS OF PREGNANCY UNLESS SPECIFICALLY DIRECTED TO DO SO BY A DOCTOR BECAUSE IT MAY CAUSE PROBLEMS IN THE UNBORN CHILD OR COMPLICATIONS DURING DELIVERY.

DRIXORAL COLD & ALLERGY 12 HOUR RELIEF
Schering-Plough HealthCare Products

Dosage Form: timed-release tablet

Active Ingredients: pseudoephedrine sulfate, dexbrompheniramine maleate

Warning: Do not exceed recommended dosage because at higher dosages, nervousness, dizziness, or sleeplessness may occur. If symptoms do not improve within 7 days or are accompanied by a fever, consult a doctor. Do not take this product if you have asthma, glaucoma, emphysema, chronic pulmonary disease, shortness of breath, difficulty in breathing, heart disease, high blood pressure, diabetes, thyroid disease or difficulty in urination due to enlargement of the prostate gland, or give this product to children under 12 years of age, unless directed by a doctor. May cause excitability especially in children. May cause drowsiness; alcohol, sedatives, and tranquilizers may increase its drowsiness effect. Avoid alcoholic beverages while taking this product. Do not take this product if you are taking sedatives or tranquilizers without first consulting your doctor. Use caution while driving a motor vehicle or operating machinery. DRUG INTERACTION PRECAUTION: Do not use this product if you are now taking a prescription monoamine oxidase inhibitor (MAOI) (certain drugs for depression, psychiatric or emotional conditions, or Parkinson's disease) or for 2 weeks after stopping the MAOI drug. If you are uncertain if your prescription drug contains an MAOI, consult a health professional before taking this product.

DRIXORAL COLD & FLU 12 HOUR RELIEF
Schering-Plough HealthCare Products

Dosage Form: timed-release tablet

Active Ingredients: pseudoephedrine sulfate, dexbrompheniramine maleate, acetaminophen

Warning: Do not exceed recommended dosage because at higher dosages, nervousness, dizziness, or sleeplessness may occur. Do not take this product for more than 7 days. If symptoms do not improve or are accompanied by fever that lasts for more than 3 days or recurs, or if new symptoms occur, consult a doctor before continuing use. If pain or fever persists, or gets worse, or if redness or swelling is present, consult a doctor. These could be signs of a serious condition. Do not take this product, if you have asthma, glaucoma, emphysema or chronic pul-

monary disease, shortness of breath, difficulty in breathing, heart disease, high blood pressure, thyroid disease, diabetes or difficulty in urination due to the enlargement of the prostate gland, or give this product to children under 12 years of age, without first consulting a doctor. May cause excitability especially in children. May cause drowsiness; alcohol, sedatives, and tranquilizers may increase its drowsiness effect. Avoid alcoholic beverages while taking this product. Do not take this product if you are taking sedatives or tranquilizers without first consulting your doctor. Use caution while driving a motor vehicle or operating machinery. Do not use with other products containing acetaminophen. DRUG INTERACTION PRECAUTION: Do not use this product if you are now taking a prescription drug for high blood pressure without first consulting your doctor or if you are now taking a prescription monoamine oxidase inhibitor (MAOI) (certain drugs for depression, psychiatric or emotional conditions, or Parkinson's disease) or for 2 weeks after stopping the MAOI drug. If you are uncertain if your prescription drug contains an MAOI, consult a health professional before taking this product.

DRIXORAL COUGH LIQUID CAPS
Schering-Plough HealthCare Products

Dosage Form: capsule

Active Ingredient: dextromethorphan hydrobromide

Warning: A persistent cough may be a sign of a serious condition. If cough persists for more than 1 week, tends to recur, or is accompanied by a fever, rash, or persistent headache consult a doctor. Do not take this product for persistent or chronic cough such as occurs with smoking, asthma, chronic bronchitis, emphysema, or if cough is accompanied by excessive phlegm (mucous) unless directed by a doctor. Do not crush or chew tablets. Swallow whole. DRUG INTERACTION PRECAUTION: Do not use this product if you are now taking a prescription monoamine oxidase inhibitor (MAOI) (certain drugs for depression, psychiatric or emotional conditions, or Parkinson's disease) or for 2 weeks after stopping the MAOI drug. If you are uncertain if your prescription drug contains an MAOI, consult a health professional before taking this product.

DRIXORAL NON-DROWSY NASAL DECONGESTANT 12 HOUR RELIEF
Schering-Plough HealthCare Products

Dosage Form: timed-release tablet

Active Ingredient: pseudoephedrine sulfate

Warning: Do not exceed recommended dosage because at higher dosages, nervousness, dizziness, or sleeplessness may occur. If symptoms do not improve within 7 days or are accompanied by a fever, consult a doctor. Do not take this product if you have heart disease, high blood pressure, diabetes, thyroid disease, or difficulty in urination due to enlargement of the prostate gland, or give this product to children under 12 years of age unless directed by a doctor. Do not crush or

chew tablets. Swallow whole. DRUG INTERACTION PRECAUTION: Do not use this product if you are now taking a prescription drug for high blood pressure without first consulting your doctor or if you are now taking a prescription monoamine oxidase inhibitor (MAOI) (certain drugs for depression, psychiatric or emotional conditions, or Parkinson's disease) or for 2 weeks after stopping the MAOI drug. If you are uncertain if your prescription drug contains an MAOI, consult a health professional before taking this product.

DRY EYE THERAPY
Bausch & Lomb
Personal Products Division

Dosage Form: drops

Active Ingredient: glycerin

Warning: To avoid contamination, do not touch tip of container to any surface. If you experience eye pain, changes in vision, continued redness or irritation of the eye, or if the condition worsens or persists for more than 72 hours, discontinue use and consult a doctor. If solution changes color or becomes cloudy, do not use.

DULCOLAX
*Ciba Self-Medication, Inc.**

Dosage Form: tablet, suppository

Active Ingredients: bisacodyl

Warning: Do not use laxative products when abdominal pain, nausea, or vomiting are present unless directed by a doctor. Restoration of normal bowel function by using this product may cause abdominal discomfort including cramps. If you have noticed a sudden change in bowel habits that persists over a period of 2 weeks, consult a doctor before using a laxative. Laxative products should not be used for a period longer than 1 week unless directed by a doctor. Rectal bleeding or failure to have a bowel movement after use of a laxative may indicate a serious condition. Discontinue use and consult a doctor. *For tablets:* Do not chew or crush. Do not give to children under 6 years of age unless directed by a doctor. Do not take this product within 1 hour after taking an antacid or milk.

DUOFILM WART REMOVER
Schering-Plough HealthCare Products

Dosage Form: liquid

Active Ingredient: salicylic acid

Warning: For external use only. Do not use this product on irritated skin, on any area that is infected or reddened, if you are a diabetic, or if you have poor blood circulation. If discomfort persists, see your doctor. Do not use on moles, birthmarks, warts with hair growing from them, genital warts, or warts on the face or mucous membranes. If product gets in the eyes, flush with water for 15 minutes. Extremely flammable. Keep away from fire or flame. Avoid inhaling vapors.

DUOPLANT PLANTAR WART REMOVER
Schering-Plough HealthCare Products

Dosage Form: gel

Active Ingredient: salicylic acid

Warning: For external use only. Do not use this product on irritated skin, on any area that is infected or reddened, if you are a diabetic, or if you have poor blood circulation. If discomfort persists, see your doctor. Do not use on moles, birthmarks, warts with hair growing from them, genital warts, or warts on the face or mucous membranes. If product gets in the eyes, flush with water for 15 minutes. Extremely flammable. Keep away from fire or flame. Cap tube tightly and store at room temperature away from heat. Avoid inhaling vapors.

DURATION 12 HOUR SPRAY
Schering-Plough HealthCare Products

Dosage Form: spray

Active Ingredient: oxymetazoline hydrochloride (HCl)

Warning: Do not exceed recommended dosage. This product may cause temporary discomfort, such as burning, stinging, sneezing, or an increase in nasal discharge. Do not use for more than 3 days. Use only as directed. Frequent or prolonged use may cause nasal congestion to recur or worsen. If symptoms persist, consult a doctor. Do not take this product if you have heart disease, high blood pressure, thyroid disease, diabetes or difficulty in urination due to enlargement of the prostate gland unless directed by a doctor. Do not use this product on a child who has heart disease, high blood pressure, thyroid disease, or diabetes unless directed by a doctor. The use of this container by more than one person may spread infection.

E

ECOTRIN MAXIMUM STRENGTH
SmithKline Beecham
Consumer Health Care, L.P.

Dosage Form: tablet

Active Ingredient: aspirin

Warning: Children and teenagers should not use this medicine for chicken pox or flu symptoms before a doctor is consulted about Reye Syndrome, a rare but serious illness reported to be associated with aspirin. Do not take for pain for more than 10 days or for fever for more than 3 days unless directed by a doctor. If pain or fever persists or gets worse, if new symptoms occur, or if redness or swelling is present, consult a doctor. These could be signs of serious illness. Do not take this product if you are allergic to aspirin, have asthma, have stomach problems (such as heartburn, upset stomach or stomach pain) that persist or recur, or if you have ulcers or bleeding problems, unless directed by a doctor. If ringing in the ears or loss of hearing occurs, consult a doctor

before taking any more of this product. Do not crush or chew tablets. Swallow whole. DRUG INTERACTION PRECAUTION: Do not use if taking a prescription drug for anticoagulation (blood thinning), diabetes, gout or arthritis unless directed by a doctor. IT IS ESPECIALLY IMPORTANT NOT TO USE ASPIRIN DURING THE LAST 3 MONTHS OF PREGNANCY UNLESS SPECIFICALLY DIRECTED TO DO SO BY A DOCTOR BECAUSE IT MAY CAUSE PROBLEMS IN THE UNBORN CHILD OR COMPLICATIONS DURING DELIVERY.

EFIDAC/24
Ciba Self-Medication, Inc.*

Dosage Form: timed-release tablet

Active Ingredient: pseudoephedrine hydrochloride (HCl)

Warning: Do not exceed recommended dosage because at higher dosages nervousness, dizziness or sleeplessness may occur. Do not take this product for more than 7 days. If symptoms do not improve or are accompanied by a fever consult a doctor. Do not take this product if you have heart disease, high blood pressure, diabetes, thyroid disease, or difficulty in urination due to enlargement of the prostate gland unless directed by a doctor. Rarely tablets of this kind may cause bowel obstruction (blockage), usually in people with severe narrowing of the bowel (esophagus, stomach or intestine). If you have had obstruction or narrowing of the bowel do not take this product without consulting your doctor. Contact your doctor if you experience persistent abdominal pain or vomiting. Do not crush or chew tablets. Swallow whole. DRUG INTERACTION PRECAUTION: Do not take this product if you are presently taking a prescription drug for high blood pressure or depression without first consulting your doctor. Do not use this product if you are now taking a prescription monoamine oxidase inhibitor (MAOI) (certain drugs for depression, psychiatric or emotional conditions, or Parkinson's disease) or for 2 weeks after stopping the MAOI drug. If you are uncertain if your prescription drug contains an MAOI, consult a health professional before taking this product.

EFIDAC 24 CHLORPHENIRAMINE
Ciba Self-Medication, Inc.*

Dosage Form: timed-release tablet

Active Ingredient: chlorpheniramine maleate

Warning: Do not exceed recommended dosage. May cause excitability, especially in children. Do not take this product, unless directed by a doctor, if you have breathing problems such as emphysema, or chronic bronchitis, or if you have glaucoma, or difficulty in urination due to enlargement of the prostate gland. May cause drowsiness; alcohol, sedatives, and tranquilizers may increase its drowsiness effect. Avoid alcoholic beverages while taking this product. Do not take this product while taking sedatives or tranquilizers without first consulting your doctor. Use caution while driving a motor vehicle or operating machinery. Rarely tablets of this kind may cause bowel

obstruction (blockage), usually in people with severe narrowing of the bowel (esophagus, stomach or intestine). If you have had obstruction or narrowing of the bowel do not take this product without consulting your doctor. Contact your doctor if you experience persistent abdominal pain or vomiting. Do not crush or chew tablets. Swallow whole.

EMETROL
Pharmacia & Upjohn, Inc.

Dosage Form: liquid

Active Ingredient: phosphoric acid, dextrose, levulose

Warning: This product contains fructose and should not be taken by persons with hereditary fructose intolerance (HFI). This product contains sugar and should not be taken by diabetics, except under the advice and supervision of a doctor. *Caution:* Not to be taken for more than 1 hour (5 doses) without consulting a doctor. If nausea continues or recurs frequently consult a doctor. For maximum effectiveness never dilute Emetrol, or drink fluids of any kind immediately before or after taking.

EQUALACTIN CHEW TABLETS
Numark Laboratories

Dosage Form: chewable tablet

Active Ingredient: polycarbophil

Warning: WARNINGS FOR CONSTIPATION: Do not use a laxative when abdominal pain, nausea, vomiting are present, unless directed by a doctor. Consult a doctor if a sudden change in bowel habit occurs or if the product has no effect within a week. Rectal bleeding or no bowel movement after the use of a laxative may indicate a serious condition. Discontinue use and consult a doctor. Do not use in children under 3 years of age unless directed by a doctor. WARNINGS FOR DIARRHEA: Chew tablets. Do not use for more than 2 days, or in the presence of fever, or in children under 3 years of age unless directed by a doctor. INTERACTION PRECAUTION: Contains calcium. Do not use if you are taking a prescription antibiotic drug containing any form of tetracycline.

EUCERIN DRY SKIN THERAPY ORIGINAL
Beiersdorf, Inc.

Dosage Form: lotion, cream

Active Ingredients: No active ingredients have been indicated by the manufacturer.

Warning: For external use only. Discontinue use if irritation occurs.

EX-LAX REGULAR STRENGTH LAXATIVE PILLS
Sandoz North American
Consumer Pharmaceuticals*

Dosage Form: tablet

Active Ingredient: yellow phenolphthalein

Warning: Do not use laxative products when abdominal pain, nausea, or vomiting are present unless directed by a doctor. Frequent or prolonged use of this or any other laxative may result in dependence on laxatives. If skin rash appears, do not use this product or any other preparation containing phenolphthalein.

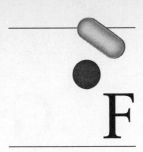

F

FEEN-A-MINT BISACODYL STIMULANT LAXATIVE
Schering-Plough HealthCare Products

Dosage Form: tablet

Active Ingredient: bisacodyl

Warning: Do not chew tablets. Do not give to children under 6 years of age, or to persons who cannot swallow without chewing, unless directed by a doctor. Do not take this product within 1 hour after taking an antacid or milk. Do not use laxative products when abdominal pain, nausea, or vomiting are present unless directed by a doctor. If you have noticed a sudden change in bowel habits that persists over a period of 2 weeks, consult a doctor before using a laxative. Laxative products should not be used for a period longer than 1 week unless directed by a doctor. Rectal bleeding or failure to have a bowel movement after use of a laxative may indicate a serious condition. Discontinue use and consult a doctor. This product may cause abdominal discomfort, faintness and cramps.

FEMSTAT 3
The Procter & Gamble Company

Dosage Form: cream

Active Ingredient: butoconazole nitrate

Warning: Do not use if you have abdominal pain, fever, or foul-smelling discharge. Contact your doctor immediately. If your infection is not gone in 3 days, you may have a condition other than a yeast infection or you may need to use more medication. Consult your doctor. If your symptoms return within 2 months or if you think you have been exposed to the human imunodefiency virus (HIV) that causes AIDS, consult your doctor immediately. Recurring infections may be a sign of pregnancy or a serious condition, such as AIDS or diabetes. Do not use this product if you are pregnant or think you may be pregnant, have diabetes, a positive HIV test or AIDS. Consult your doctor. Do not rely on condoms or diaphragms to prevent sexually transmitted diseases or pregnancy while using this product. This product may damage condoms and diaphragms and may cause them to fail. Use another method of birth control to prevent pregnancy while using this product. Do not use tampons while using this medicine. Do not use in girls under 12 years of age.

FIBERALL PREMIUM PSYLLIUM FIBER
Ciba Self-Medication, Inc.[*]

Dosage Form: powder

Active Ingredient: psyllium hydrophilic mucilloid

Warning: Do not use laxative products when abdominal pain, nausea, or vomiting are present unless directed by a doctor. If you have noticed a sudden change in bowel habits that persists over a period of 2 weeks, consult a doctor before using a laxative. Laxative products should not be used for a period longer than 1 week unless directed by a doctor. Discontinue use and consult a doctor if rectal bleeding or failure to have a bowel movement occurs after using any laxative product. With any natural grain product, inhaled or ingested powder may cause an allergic reaction in individuals sensitive to it. TAKING THIS PRODUCT WITHOUT ADEQUATE FLUID MAY CAUSE IT TO SWELL AND BLOCK YOUR THROAT OR ESOPHAGUS AND MAY CAUSE CHOKING. DO NOT TAKE THIS PRODUCT IF YOU HAVE DIFFICULTY IN SWALLOWING. IF YOU EXPERIENCE CHEST PAIN, VOMITING, OR DIFFICULTY IN SWALLOWING OR BREATHING AFTER TAKING THIS PRODUCT SEEK IMMEDIATE MEDICAL ATTENTION.

FIBERCON
Lederle Consumer Health

Dosage Form: tablet

Active Ingredient: calcium polycarbophil

Warning: Any sudden change in bowel habits may indicate a more serious condition than constipation. Consult your doctor if symptoms such as nausea, vomiting, abdominal pain or rectal bleeding occur or if this product has no effect in 1 week. For chronic or continued constipation consult your doctor. DRUG INTERACTION PRECAUTION: Contains calcium. If you are taking any form of tetracycline antibiotic, this product should be taken at least 1 hour before or 2 hours after you have taken the antibiotic. TAKING THIS PRODUCT WITHOUT ADEQUATE FLUID MAY CAUSE IT TO SWELL AND BLOCK YOUR THROAT OR ESOPHAGUS AND MAY CAUSE CHOKING. DO NOT TAKE THIS PRODUCT IF YOU HAVE DIFFICULTY IN SWALLOWING. IF YOU EXPERIENCE CHEST PAIN, VOMITING, OR DIFFICULTY IN SWALLOWING OR BREATHING AFTER TAKING THIS PRODUCT SEEK IMMEDIATE MEDICAL ATTENTION.

FISHERMAN'S FRIEND EXTRA STRENGTH
Bristol-Myers Products

Dosage Form: lozenge

Active Ingredients: menthol

Warning: A persistent cough may be a sign of a serious condition. If cough or sore throat is severe, persists for more than 2 days, tends to recur, or is accompanied by a fever, headache, rash, swelling, nausea or vomiting, consult a doctor. Do not take this product for persistent or chronic cough such as occurs with smoking, asthma, emphysema, or if cough is accompanied by excessive phlegm (mucous) unless directed by a doctor. Do not exceed recommended dosage.

FLEET GLYCERIN SUPPOSITORIES ADULT SIZE
C. B. Fleet Company, Inc.

Dosage Form: suppository

Active Ingredient: glycerin

Warning: May cause rectal discomfort or a burning sensation. For rectal use only. Do not use laxative products when abdominal pain, nausea, or vomiting are present unless directed by a doctor. If you have noticed a sudden change in bowel habits that persists over a period of 2 weeks, consult a doctor before using a laxative. Laxative products should not be used for a period longer than 1 week unless directed by a doctor. Rectal bleeding or failure to have a bowel movement after use of a laxative may indicate a serious condition. Discontinue use and consult a doctor.

FLEET GLYCERIN SUPPOSITORIES CHILD SIZE
C. B. Fleet Company, Inc.

Dosage Form: suppository

Active Ingredient: glycerin

Warning: May cause rectal discomfort or a burning sensation. For rectal use only. Do not use laxative products when abdominal pain, nausea, or vomiting are present unless directed by a doctor. If you have noticed a sudden change in bowel habits that persists over a period of 2 weeks, consult a doctor before using a laxative. Laxative products should not be used for a period longer than 1 week unless directed by a doctor. Rectal bleeding or failure to have a bowel movement after use of a laxative may indicate a serious condition. Discontinue use and consult a doctor.

FLEET PHOSPHO-SODA BUFFERED SALINE ORAL LAXATIVE
C. B. Fleet Company, Inc.

Dosage Form: liquid

Active Ingredients: monobasic sodium phosphate, dibasic sodium phosphate

Warning: Do not exceed recommended dose unless directed by a doctor. Serious side effects may result from excessive dosage. Do not use laxative products when abdominal pain, nausea, or vomiting are present unless directed by a doctor. If you have noticed a sudden change in bowel habits that persists over a period of 2 weeks, consult a doctor before using a laxative. Rectal bleeding or failure to have a bowel movement after use of a laxative may indicate a serious condition. Discontinue use and consult a doctor. Laxative products should not be used for a period longer than 1 week unless directed by a doctor. Do not use this product if you are on a sodium restricted diet or if you have kidney disease unless directed by a doctor. If foil imprinted with safety seal is broken or missing do not use.

FLEET READY-TO-USE ENEMA
C. B. Fleet Company, Inc.

Dosage Form: enema

Active Ingredients: monobasic sodium phosphate, dibasic sodium phosphate

Warning: Do not use laxative products when abdominal pain, nausea, or vomiting are present unless directed by a doctor. If you have noticed a sudden change in bowel habits that persists over a period of 2 weeks, consult a doctor before using a laxative. Laxative products should not be used for a period longer than 1 week unless directed by a doctor. Rectal bleeding or failure to have a bowel movement after use of a laxative may indicate a serious condition. Discontinue use and consult a doctor. Do not use this product if you are on a sodium restricted diet or if you have kidney disease unless directed by a doctor.

FLETCHER'S CASTORIA
Mentholatum Company, Inc.

Dosage Form: liquid

Active Ingredient: senna concentrate

Warning: Do not use laxative products when abdominal pain, nausea, or vomiting are present unless directed by a doctor. If you have noticed a sudden change in bowel habits that persists over a period of 2 weeks, consult a doctor before using a laxative. Laxative products should not be used for a period longer than 1 week unless directed by a doctor. Rectal bleeding or failure to have a bowel movement after use of a laxative may indicate a serious condition. Discontinue use and consult a doctor.

FLETCHER'S CHERRY THE CHILDREN'S LAXATIVE
Mentholatum Company, Inc.

Dosage Form: suspension

Active Ingredient: yellow phenolphthalein

Warning: Do not use laxative products when abdominal pain, nausea, or vomiting are present unless directed by a doctor. If you have noticed a sudden change in bowel habits that persists over a period of 2 weeks, consult a doctor before using a laxative. Laxative products should not be used for a period longer than 1 week unless directed by a doctor. Rectal bleeding or failure to have a bowel movement after use of a laxative may indicate a serious condition. Discontinue use and consult a doctor. If a skin rash appears, do not use this product or any other preparation containing phenolphthalein.

FLEX-ALL 454 MAXIMUM STRENGTH
Chattem, Inc.

Dosage Form: gel

Active Ingredients: menthol

Warning: For external use only. Use only as directed. Avoid contact with eyes and mucous membranes. If skin redness or irritation develops, or pain lasts for more than 10 days, or clears up and occurs again within a few days, discontinue use and consult a doctor. If prone to allergic reaction to aspirin or salicylates, consult a doctor before using. Do not apply to wounds, or to damaged, broken (open) or irritated skin. Do not bandage tightly. Do not use with a heating pad.

FOILLE MEDICATED FIRST AID
Blistex Inc.

Dosage Form: ointment, aerosol

Active Ingredients: benzocaine, chloroxylenol

Warning: Do not use in eyes. In case of deep or puncture wounds, or serious burns, consult a doctor. If condition worsens, if a rash or irritation develops or if symptoms persist, discontinue use of this product and consult a doctor. Not for prolonged use. Certain persons can develop allergic reactions to ingredients in this product. Do not use this product if you have a history of allergy to local anesthetics such as procaine, butacaine, benzocaine, or other "caine" anesthetics.

FOSTEX 10% BENZOYL PEROXIDE VANISHING GEL
Bristol-Myers Products

Dosage Form: gel

Active Ingredient: benzoyl peroxide

Warning: For external use only. Keep away from eyes, lips, mouth and sensitive areas of the neck. If contact with eyes occurs, flush thoroughly with water. Using other topical acne medications at the same time or immediately following use of this product may increase dryness or irritation of the skin. If this occurs only one medication should be used unless directed by a doctor. Do not use this medication if you have very sensitive skin or if you are sensitive to benzoyl peroxide. This product may cause irritation, characterized by redness, burning, itching, peeling or possibly swelling. More frequent use or higher concentrations may aggravate such irritation. Mild irritation may be reduced by using the product less frequently or in a lower concentration. If irritation becomes severe, discontinue use; if irritation still continues consult a doctor. This product may bleach hair or dyed fabrics.

FOSTEX ACNE MEDICATION CLEANSING BAR
Bristol-Myers Products

Dosage Form: cleansing bar

Active Ingredient: salicylic acid

Warning: For external use only. Avoid contact with eyes. If contact occurs, flush thoroughly with water. Using other topical acne medications at the same time or immediately following use of this product may increase dryness or irritation of the skin. If this occurs, only one medication should be used unless directed by a doctor.

FREEZONE CORN AND CALLUS REMOVER
Whitehall-Robins Healthcare

Dosage Form: liquid

Active Ingredient: salicylic acid

Warning: For external use only. Do not use this product on irritated skin, or any area that is infected or reddened, if you are a diabetic, or if you have poor blood circulation. If discomfort persists, see a doctor or podiatrist. If product gets into eye, flush with water for 15 minutes.

GAS-X
Sandoz North American Consumer Pharmaceuticals*

Dosage Form: chewable tablet

Active Ingredient: simethicone

Warning: If symptoms persist, contact your doctor.

GAVISCON EXTRA STRENGTH ANTACID
SmithKline Beecham Consumer Health Care, L.P.

Dosage Form: liquid, chewable tablet

Active Ingredients: aluminum hydroxide, magnesium carbonate

Warning: Do not take more than 16 teaspoonfuls in a 24-hour period, or 16 teaspoonfuls daily for a 2 week period. May have laxative effect. Do not use this product if you have a kidney disease, except under the advice and supervision of a doctor. Do not use this product if you are on a sodium restricted diet. Each tablespoon of GAVISCON Liquid contains approximately 0.9mEq. sodium. DRUG INTERACTION PRECAUTION: Antacids may interact with certain prescription drugs. If you are presently taking a prescription drug, do not take this product without checking with your doctor or other health professional.

GLY-OXIDE
SmithKline Beecham Consumer Health Care, L.P.

Dosage Form: liquid

Active Ingredient: carbamide peroxide

Warning: Severe or present oral inflammation, denture irritation, or gingivitis may be serious. Do not use this product for more than 7 days unless directed by a dentist or doctor. If sore mouth symptoms do not improve; if irritation, pain, or redness, persists or worsens; or if swelling, rash or fever develops, discontinue use of product and see your dentist or doctor promptly.

GYNE-LOTRIMIN 3
Schering-Plough HealthCare Products

Dosage Form: cream

Active Ingredient: clotrimazole

Warning: Do not use if you have abdominal pain, fever, or foul-smelling discharge. Contact your doctor immediately. If your symptoms do not improve in 3 days, or if your infection is not gone in 7 days, you may have a condition other than a yeast infection. Consult your doctor. If your symptoms return within 2 months or if you have infections that do not clear up easily with proper treatment, consult your doctor. You could be pregnant or there could be a serious underlying medical cause for your infections, including diabetes, or a damaged immune system (including damage from infection with HIV—the virus that causes AIDS). Do not use during pregnancy except under the advice and supervision of a doctor. Do not use tampons while using this medication. Do not use in children less than 12 years of age.

GYNE-MOISTRIN
Schering-Plough HealthCare Products

Dosage Form: gel

Active Ingredients: No active ingredients have been indicated by the manufacturer.

Warning: Do not use as a contraceptive.

HALEY'S M-O LUBRICANT LAXATIVE
Bayer Corporation,
Consumer Care Division

Dosage Form: emulsion

Active Ingredient: mineral oil

Warning: Do not use laxative products when abdominal pain, nausea, vomiting or kidney disease are present unless directed by a doctor. If you have noticed a sudden change in bowel habits that persists over a period of 2 weeks, consult a doctor before using a laxative. Laxative products should not be used for a period longer than 1 week unless directed by a doctor. Rectal bleeding or failure to have a bowel movement after use of a laxative may indicate a serious condition. Discontinue use and consult a doctor. Do not administer to children under 6 years of age, to pregnant women, to bedridden patients or to persons with difficulty in swallowing. Do not take with meals. DRUG INTERACTION PRECAUTION: Do not take this product if you are presently taking a stool softener laxative, unless directed by a doctor.

HALLS MENTHOL/COUGH SUPPRESSANT DROPS
Warner-Lambert

Dosage Form: lozenge

Active Ingredient: menthol

Warning: A persistent cough may be a sign of a serious condition. If cough is severe, persists for more than 1 week, tends to recur, or is accompanied by a fever, headache, rash, swelling, nausea or vomiting, consult a doctor. Do not take this product for persistent or chronic cough such as occurs with smoking, asthma, emphysema, or if cough is accompanied by excessive phlegm (mucous) unless directed by a doctor. If sore throat is severe, persists

for more than 2 days, tends to recur, or is accompanied by a fever, headache, rash, swelling, nausea or vomiting, consult a doctor. Do not exceed recommended dosage.

HEAD & SHOULDERS DANDRUFF SHAMPOO
The Procter & Gamble Company

Dosage Form: shampoo

Active Ingredient: pyrithione zinc

Warning: For external use only. Avoid contact with the eyes. If contact occurs, rinse eyes thoroughly with water. If condition worsens or does not improve after regular use of this product as directed, consult a doctor.

HEET PAIN RELIEVING LINIMENT
Whitehall-Robins Healthcare

Dosage Form: liniment

Active Ingredients: methyl salicylate, camphor, capsaicin

Warning: For external use only. Use only as directed. Avoid contact with eyes and mucous membranes. If skin redness or irritation develops, if condition worsens, or does not improve within 7 days, or clears up and occurs again within a few days, discontinue use and consult a doctor. If prone to allergic reaction to aspirin or salicylates, consult a doctor before using. Do not apply to wounds, or to damaged, broken (open) or irritated skin. Do not bandage tightly. Do not apply external heat or hot water when using this product as this may cause skin burns. Extremely flammable. Keep away from fire or flame. Avoid smoking during application and until product is dried. If you are a diabetic or have impaired circulation, use Heet only on the advice of a doctor. Let product dry thoroughly before permitting contact with clothing.

HEMORID FOR WOMEN HEMORRHOIDAL CREME
Pfizer Inc., Consumer Care Group

Dosage Form: cream, ointment

Active Ingredients: pramoxine hydrochloride (HCl), phenylephrine hydrochloride (HCl), petrolatum, mineral oil

Warning: Do not apply to large areas of the body. If condition worsens or pain persists for more than 7 days, or clears up and occurs again within a few days, discontinue use and consult a doctor. If the symptom being treated does not subside or if redness, irritation, swelling, pain or other symptoms develop or increase, discontinue use and consult a doctor. Do not exceed recommended dosage, unless directed by a doctor. In case of bleeding, consult a doctor promptly. Do not put this product into the rectum by using fingers or any mechanical device or applicator. Certain persons can develop allergic reactions to ingredients in this product. Do not use in the eyes or nose. Do not use this product if you have heart disease, high blood pressure, thyroid disease, diabetes, or difficulty in urination due to the enlargement of the prostate gland unless directed by a doctor. DRUG INTERACTION PRECAUTION: Do not use this product if you are presently taking a prescription drug for high blood pressure or depression, without first consulting your doctor.

HOLD DM
Menley & James Laboratories, Inc.

Dosage Form: lozenge

Active Ingredient: dextromethorphan hydrobromide

Warning: A persistent cough may be a sign of a serious condition. If cough persists for more than 1 week, tends to recur, or is accompanied by a fever, rash or persistent headache, consult a doctor. Do not take this product for persistent or chronic cough such as occurs with smoking, asthma, emphysema, or if cough is accompanied by excessive phlegm (mucous) unless directed by a doctor. DRUG INTERACTION PRECAUTION: Do not use this product if you are now taking a prescription monoamine oxidase inhibitor (MAOI) (certain drugs for depression, psychiatric or emotional conditions, or Parkinson's disease) or for 2 weeks after stopping the MAOI drug. If you are uncertain if your prescription drug contains an MAOI, consult a health professional before taking this product.

HYPOTEARS
Ciba Vision Ophthalmics

Dosage Form: drops

Active Ingredients: polyvinyl alcohol, polyethylene glycol 400

Warning: To avoid contamination, do not touch tip of container to any surface. Replace cap after usage. If you experience eye pain, changes in vision, continued redness or irritation of the eye, or if your condition worsens or persists for more than 72 hours, discontinue use and consult a doctor. If the solution changes color or becomes cloudy, do not use. Do not use this product if you are allergic to any of its ingredients.

ICY HOT
Chattem, Inc.

Dosage Form: cream, ointment, stick

Active Ingredients: methyl salicylate, menthol

Warning: For external use only. Use only as directed. Avoid contact with eyes and mucous membranes. If skin redness or irritation develops, or pain lasts for more than 10 days, or clears up and occurs again within a few days, discontinue use and consult a doctor. If prone to allergic reaction to aspirin or salicylates, consult a doctor before using. Do not apply to wounds, or to damaged, broken (open) or irritated skin. Do not bandage tightly. Do not use with a heating pad.

IMODIUM A-D
McNeil Consumer Products Company

Dosage Form: caplet, liquid

Active Ingredient: loperamide hydrochloride (HCl)

Warning: Do not use for more than 2 days unless directed by a doctor. Do not use if diarrhea is accompanied by a high fever (greater than 101°F), or if blood or mucous is present in the stool, or if you have had a rash or other allergic reaction to loperamide hydrochloride. If you are taking antibiotics or have a history of liver disease, consult a doctor before using this product.

IONIL
Galderma Laboratories, Inc.

Dosage Form: shampoo

Active Ingredient: salicylic acid

Warning: For external use only. Avoid contact with the eyes. If contact occurs, rinse eyes thoroughly with water. If condition worsens or does not improve after regular use of this product as directed, consult a doctor. If condition covers large area of the body, consult your doctor before using this product.

IONIL T PLUS
Galderma Laboratories, Inc.

Dosage Form: shampoo

Active Ingredient: coal tar

Warning: For external use only. Avoid contact with the eyes. If contact occurs, rinse eyes thoroughly with water. If condition worsens or does not improve after regular use of this product as directed, consult a doctor. Use caution in exposing skin to sunlight after applying this product. It may increase tendency to sunburn for up to 24 hours after application. Do not use for prolonged periods without consulting a doctor. Do not use this product with other forms of psoriasis therapy, such as ultraviolet radiation or prescription drugs, unless directed by a doctor.

IVAREST 8-HOUR RELIEF MEDICATED CREAM
Blistex Inc.

Dosage Form: cream

Active Ingredients: diphenhydramine hydrochloride (HCl), calamine

Warning: For external use only. Avoid contact with the eyes. If condition worsens, does not improve within 7 days, or if symptoms persist for more than 7 days or clear up and occur again within a few days, discontinue use and consult a doctor. Ivarest may stain certain fabrics, so avoid contact with clothing. Do not use with any other drugs containing diphenhydramine while using this product.

J

JERGENS ADVANCED THERAPY DRY SKIN CARE
Andrew Jergens Company

Dosage Form: lotion

Active Ingredient: No active ingredients have been indicated by the manufacturer.

Warning: No warnings have been indicated by the manufacturer.

JOHNSON'S DIAPER RASH OINTMENT
Johnson & Johnson Consumer Products, Inc.

Dosage Form: ointment

Active Ingredients: petrolatum, zinc oxide

Warning: For external use only. Avoid contact with eyes. If condition worsens, or does not improve within 7 days, consult your doctor.

K

K-Y JELLY
Johnson & Johnson Consumer Products, Inc.

Dosage Form: jelly

Active Ingredients: No active ingredients have been indicated by the manufacturer.

Warning: Do not use as a contraceptive.

KANK-A PROFESSIONAL STRENGTH MOUTH SORE MEDICATION
Blistex Inc.

Dosage Form: liquid

Active Ingredients: benzocaine, benzoin tincture compound

Warning: Do not use this product for more than 7 days unless directed by a dentist or doctor. If sore mouth symptoms do not improve; if irritation, pain, or redness, persists or worsens; or if swelling, rash or fever develops, discontinue use of this product and see your dentist or doctor promptly. Do not exceed recommended dosage. Do not use this product if you have a history of allergy to local anesthetics such as procaine, butacaine, benzocaine, or other "caine" anesthetics. Avoid contact with the eyes. Avoid contact with clothing and

household/furniture surfaces to prevent possible staining. This product is a personal care item, and should be used by one individual only.

KAOPECTATE
Pharmacia & Upjohn, Inc.

Dosage Form: caplet, liquid

Active Ingredient: attapulgite

Warning: Do not use for more than 2 days unless directed by a doctor. Do not use if diarrhea is accompanied by a fever, or if blood or mucus is present in the stool. Do not use in infants or children under 3 years of age unless directed by a doctor. If you are taking a prescription medicine, consult your doctor before taking this product.

KERI ORIGINAL
Bristol-Myers Products

Dosage Form: lotion

Active Ingredient: No active ingredients have been indicared by the manufacturer.

Warning: For external use only.

KERICORT 10
Bristol-Myers Products

Dosage Form: cream

Active Ingredient: hydrocortisone

Warning: For external use only. Avoid contact with the eyes. If condition worsens, or if symptoms persist for more than 7 days or clear up and occur again within a few days, stop use of this product and do not begin use of any other hydrocortizone product unless you have consulted a doctor. Do not use for the treatment of diaper rash. Consult a doctor.

KONDREMUL
Ciba Self-Medication, Inc.*

Dosage Form: emulsion

Active Ingredients: mineral oil

Warning: Do not take with meals. Do not administer to children under 6 years of age, to pregnant women, to bedridden patients or to persons with difficulty swallowing. Do not use this product when abdominal pain, nausea or vomiting are present, unless directed by a doctor. Laxative products should not be used for a period longer than 1 week unless directed by a doctor. If you have noticed a sudden change in bowel habits that persists over a period of 2 weeks, consult a doctor before using a laxative. Rectal bleeding or failure to have a bowel movement after use of a laxative may indicate a serious condition. Discontinue use and consult a doctor. DRUG INTERACTION PRECAUTION: Do not take this product if you are presently taking a stool softener laxative.

KONSYL PSYLLIUM HYDROPHILIC MUCILLOID
Konsyl Pharmaceuticals, Inc.

Dosage Form: powder

Active Ingredient: psyllium hydrophilic mucilloid

Warning: Do not use laxative products when abdominal pain, nausea, or vomiting are present unless directed by a doctor. If you have noticed a sudden change in bowel habits that persists over a period of 2 weeks, consult a doctor before using a laxative. Rectal bleeding or failure to have a bowel movement after use of a laxative may indicate a serious condition. Discontinue use and consult a doctor. CAUTION: Ingested or inhaled psyllium powder may cause an allergic reaction in individuals sensitive to psyllium. TAKING THIS PRODUCT WITHOUT ADEQUATE FLUID MAY CAUSE IT TO SWELL AND BLOCK YOUR THROAT OR ESOPHAGUS AND MAY CAUSE CHOKING. DO NOT TAKE THIS PRODUCT IF YOU HAVE DIFFICULTY IN SWALLOWING. IF YOU EXPERIENCE CHEST PAIN, VOMITING, OR DIFFICULTY IN SWALLOWING OR BREATHING AFTER TAKING THIS PRODUCT SEEK IMMEDIATE MEDICAL ATTENTION.

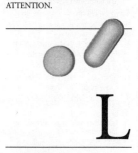

L

LANACANE MAXIMUM STRENGTH SPRAY MEDICATION
Combe, Inc.

Dosage Form: spray

Active Ingredients: aloe, benzocaine

Warning: For external use only. Do not spray into eyes, rectal or vaginal areas. Not for deep puncture wounds or serious burns. If condition worsens, if a rash or irritation develops, if symptoms persist for more than 7 days or clear up and occur again within a few days, discontinue use of this product and consult a doctor. Certain persons can develop allergic reactions to ingredients in this product. Do not use this product if you have a history of allergy to local anesthetics such as procaine, butacaine, benzocaine, or other "caine" anesthetics. Contents under pressure. Do not puncture or incinerate container or expose to heat or temperature above 120°F. Flammable mixture; do not use near fire or throw into fire. Use only as directed. Intentional misuse by deliberately concentrating and inhaling the contents can be harmful or fatal.

LANACORT 10
Combe, Inc.

Dosage Form: cream, ointment

Active Ingredient: hydrocortisone

Warning: For external use only. Avoid contact with the eyes. If condition worsens, or if symptoms persist for more than 7 days or clear up and occur again within a few days, stop use of this product and do not begin use of any other hydrocortisone product unless you have consulted a doctor. Do not use for the treatment of diaper rash. Consult a doctor. Do not use if you have a vaginal discharge. Consult a doctor.

LIQUIFILM TEARS LUBRICANT OPHTHALMIC SOLUTION
Allergan, Inc.

Dosage Form: drops

Active Ingredients: polyvinyl alcohol

Warning: To avoid contamination, do not touch tip of container to any surface. Replace cap after using. If you experience eye pain, changes in vision, continued redness or irritation of the eye, or if the condition worsens or persists for more than 72 hours, discontinue use and consult a doctor. If solution changes color or becomes cloudy, do not use.

LOTRIMIN ANTIFUNGAL AF
Schering-Plough HealthCare Products

Dosage Form: cream, solution, lotion

Active Ingredient: clotrimazole

Warning: For external use only. Do not use on children under 2 years of age unless directed by a doctor. Avoid contact with the eyes. If irritation occurs or if there is no improvement within 4 weeks (for athlete's foot or ringworm) or within 2 weeks (for jock itch), discontinue use and consult a doctor or pharmacist.

Dosage Form: spray powder, spray liquid

Active Ingredient: miconazole nitrate

Warning: For external use only. Do not use on children under 2 years of age unless directed by a doctor. If irritation occurs or if there is no improvement within 4 weeks (for athlete's foot or ringworm) or within 2 weeks (for jock itch), discontinue use and consult a doctor or pharmacist. Avoid inhaling. Avoid contact with the eyes and other mucous membranes. Contents under pressure. Do not puncture or incinerate. Flammable mixture, do not use while smoking or near fire or flame. Do not expose to heat or temperatures above 49°C (120°F). Use only as directed. Intentional misuse by deliberately concentrating and inhaling the contents can be harmful or fatal.

LUBRICATING GEL
Lake Pharmaceutical

Dosage Form: gel

Active Ingredients: No active ingredients have been indicated by the manufacturer.

Warning: Do not use if seals are broken or missing.

LUBRIDERM SKIN THERAPY MOISTURIZING LOTION
Warner Wellcome Consumer

Dosage Form: cream

Active Ingredient: No active ingredients have been indicated by the manufacturer.

Warning: For external use only.

M

MAALOX ANTI-DIARRHEAL
Ciba Self-Medication, Inc.*

Dosage Form: caplet

Active Ingredient: loperamide hydrochloride (HCl)

Warning: Do not use for more than 2 days unless directed by a doctor. Do not use if diarrhea is accompanied by a high fever (greater than 101°F), or if blood or mucous is present in the stool, or if you have had a rash or other allergic reaction to loperamide hydrochloride. If you are taking antibiotics or have a history of liver disease, consult a doctor before using this product.

MAALOX ANTI-GAS REGULAR STRENGTH
Ciba Self-Medication, Inc.*

Dosage Form: tablet

Active Ingredient: simethicone

Warning: If symptoms persist, contact your doctor.

MAALOX EXTRA STRENGTH ANTACID/ANTI-GAS
Ciba Self-Medication, Inc.*

Dosage Form: suspension

Active Ingredients: magnesium hydroxide, dried aluminum, simethicone

Warning: Do not take more than 12 tablespoonfuls in a 24 hour period or use the maximum dosage of this product for more than 2 weeks. Do not use this product if you have kidney disease, except under the advice and supervision of a doctor. DRUG INTERACTION PRECAUTION: Antacids may interact with certain prescription drugs. If you are presently taking a prescription drug, do not take this product without checking with your doctor or other health professional.

MAALOX HEARTBURN RELIEF
Ciba Self-Medication, Inc.*

Dosage Form: suspension

Active Ingredients: aluminum hydroxide, magnesium carbonate

Warning: Do not take more than 16 teaspoonfuls in a 24-hour period or use the maximum dosage of this product for more than 2 weeks. Do not use this product if you have a kidney disease, except under the advice and supervision of a doctor. DRUG INTERACTION PRECAUTION: Antacids may interact with certain prescription drugs. If you are presently taking a prescription drug, do not take this product without checking with your doctor or other health professional.

MAREZINE
Martin Himmel, Inc.

Dosage Form: tablet

Active Ingredient: cyclizine hydrochloride (HCl)

Warning: Do not give to children under 6 years of age unless directed by a doctor. Do not take this product if you have asthma, glaucoma, emphysema, chronic pulmonary disease, shortness of breath, difficulty in breathing, or difficulty in urination due to enlargement of the prostate gland, unless directed by a doctor. May cause drowsiness; alcohol, sedatives, and tranquilizers may increase its drowsiness effect. Avoid alcoholic beverages while taking this product. Do not take this product if you are taking sedatives or tranquilizers without first consulting your doctor. Use caution when driving a motor vehicle or operating machinery. Not for frequent or prolonged use, except on advice of a doctor.

MEDIPLAST
Beiersdorf, Inc.

Dosage Form: plaster pad

Active Ingredient: salicylic acid

Warning: For external use only. Do not use this product on irritated, infected, or reddened skin or if you are a diabetic or have circulatory impairments. If discomfort persists, see your doctor. Do not use on moles, birthmarks, warts with hair growing from them, genital warts, or warts on the face or mucous membranes.

METAMUCIL SMOOTH TEXTURE
The Procter & Gamble Company

Dosage Form: powder

Active Ingredient: psyllium hydrophilic mucilloid

Warning: Do not use this product when abdominal pain, nausea or vomiting are present unless directed by a doctor. If you have noticed a sudden change in bowel habits that persists over a period of 2 weeks, or rectal bleeding, consult a doctor as it may be a sign of a serious medical condition. If constipation persists for longer than 1 week, consult your doctor. This could be a sign of a serious medical condition. May cause allergic reaction in people sensitive to inhaled or ingested psyllium. TAKING THIS PRODUCT WITHOUT ADEQUATE FLUID MAY CAUSE IT TO SWELL AND BLOCK YOUR THROAT OR ESOPHAGUS AND MAY CAUSE CHOKING. DO NOT TAKE THIS PRODUCT IF YOU HAVE DIFFICULTY IN SWALLOWING. IF YOU EXPERIENCE CHEST PAIN, VOMITING, OR DIFFICULTY IN SWALLOWING OR BREATHING AFTER TAKING THIS PRODUCT SEEK IMMEDIATE MEDICAL ATTENTION.

MICATIN
*Johnson & Johnson
Consumer Products, Inc.*

Dosage Form: cream, powder, spray powder, liquid spray

Active Ingredient: miconazole nitrate

Warning: For external use only. Do not use on children under 2 years of age unless directed by a doctor. Avoid contact with the eyes. If irritation

occurs or if there is no improvement within 4 weeks (for athlete's foot or ringworm) or within 2 weeks (for jock itch), discontinue use and consult a doctor or pharmacist. *For spray powder and spray liquid:* Avoid inhaling. Avoid contact with the eyes and other mucous membranes. Contents under pressure. Do not puncture or incinerate. Flammable mixture, do not use while smoking or near fire or flame. Do not expose to heat or temperatures above 49°C (120°F). Use only as directed. Intentional misuse by deliberately concentrating and inhaling the contents can be harmful or fatal.

MIDOL IB CRAMP RELIEF FORMULA
*Bayer Corporation,
Consumer Care Division*

Dosage Form: tablet

Active Ingredient: ibuprofen

Warning: Do not take for pain for more than 10 days unless directed by a doctor. If pain persists or gets worse or if new symptoms occur, consult a doctor. These could be signs of a serious illness. If you are under a doctor's care for any serious condition, consult a doctor before taking this product. As with aspirin and acetaminophen, if you have any condition which requires you to take prescription drugs or if you have had any problems or serious side effects from taking any non-prescription pain reliever, do not take this product without first discussing it with your doctor. If you experience any symptoms which are unusual or seem unrelated to the condition for which you took ibuprofen, consult a doctor before taking any more of it. Although ibuprofen is indicated for the same conditions as aspirin and acetaminophen, it should not be taken with them except under a doctor's direction. Do not combine this product with any other ibuprofen-containing product. IT IS ESPECIALLY IMPORTANT NOT TO USE ASPIRIN DURING THE LAST 3 MONTHS OF PREGNANCY UNLESS SPECIFICALLY DIRECTED TO DO SO BY A DOCTOR BECAUSE IT MAY CAUSE PROBLEMS IN THE UNBORN CHILD OR COMPLICATIONS DURING DELIVERY.

MOIST AGAIN
Lake Consumer

Dosage Form: gel

Active Ingredients: No active ingredients have been indicated by the manufacturer.

Warning: Keep out of eyes and ears. Is not a contraceptive.

MOISTURE DROPS
*Bausch & Lomb
Personal Products Division*

Dosage Form: drops

Active Ingredients: hydroxypropyl methylcellulose, glycerin, povidone

Warning: To avoid contamination, do not touch tip of container to any surface. Replace cap after using. If you experience eye pain, changes in vision, continued redness or irritation of the eye, or if the condition worsens or persists for more than 72 hours, discontinue use and consult a doctor. If solution changes color or becomes cloudy, do not use. Remove contact

lenses before using. Store at room temperature. Use before expiration date marked on the carton and bottle.

MOISTUREL SKIN PROTECTANT LOTION
Westwood-Squibb Pharmaceuticals

Dosage Form: lotion, cream

Active Ingredient: dimethicone

Warning: For external use only. Avoid contact with eyes or areas where skin is inflamed or cracked. Discontinue use if signs of irritation occur.

MONISTAT 7
*Advanced Care Products,
Division of Ortho Pharmaceutical
Corporation*

Dosage Form: cream, suppository

Active Ingredient: miconazole nitrate

Warning: Do not use Monistat 7 vaginal cream or suppositories if you have any of the following signs and symptoms. Also if they occur while using Monistat 7 vaginal cream or suppositories stop using this product and contact your doctor right away, you may have a more serious illness. Do not use if you have abdominal pain, back pain or pain in either shoulder, a fever (higher than 100°F orally), or foul-smelling discharge. If your symptoms do not improve in 3 days, or if your infection is not gone in 7 days, you may have a condition other than a yeast infection. Consult your doctor. If your symptoms return within 2 months or if you have infections that do not clear up easily with proper treatment, consult your doctor. You could be pregnant or there could be a serious underlying medical cause for your infections, including diabetes, or a damaged immune system (including damage from infection with HIV—the virus that causes AIDS). The cream contains mineral oil which may weaken latex in condoms or in diaphragms. The suppositories contain hydrogenated vegetable oil which may weaken latex in condoms or in diaphragms. Do not rely on condoms or diaphragms to prevent sexually transmitted diseases or pregnancy while using this product. Do not use tampons while using this medication. Do not use in girls less that 12 years of age.

MOTRIN CHILDREN'S
McNeil Consumer Products Company

Dosage Form: suspension

Active Ingredient: ibuprofen

Warning: ASPIRIN SENSITIVE CHILDREN: This product contains no aspirin, but may cause a severe reaction in people allergic to aspirin. Do not take this product if your child has had an allergic reaction to aspirin such as asthma, swelling, shock or hives. *Call your doctor if:* Your child is under a doctor's care for any serious condition or is taking any other drug. Your child has problems or serious side effects from taking fever reducers or pain relievers. Your child does not get any relief within 1 day (24 hours) of treatment or if pain or fever gets worse. Redness or swelling is present in the painful area. Sore throat is severe, lasts for more than 2 days, or occurs with fever, headache, rash, nausea, or vomiting. Any new symptoms appear. *Do not use:* With any other product that contains ibuprofen, aspirin, naproxin sodium, or acetaminophen. For more than 3 days for fever or pain unless directed by a doctor. For stomach pain unless directed by a doctor. If your child is dehydrated (significant fluid loss) due to continued vomiting, diarrhea or lack of fluid intake. If imprinted plastic bottle wrap or imprinted foil inner seal is broken. If stomach upset occurs while taking this product, give with food or milk. If stomach upset gets worse or lasts, call your doctor.

MOTRIN IB
Pharmacia & Upjohn, Inc.

Dosage Form: gelcap, tablet

Active Ingredient: ibuprofen

Warning: ASPIRIN SENSITIVE PATIENTS: Do not take this product if you have had a severe allergic reaction to aspirin, e.g.—asthma, swelling, shock or hives, because even though this product contains no aspirin or salicylates, cross-reactions may occur in patients allergic to aspirin. Do not take this product for pain for more than 10 days or for fever for more than 3 days unless directed by a doctor. If pain or fever persists or gets worse, if new symptoms occur, or if redness or swelling is present, consult a doctor. These could be signs of serious illness. If you are under a doctor's care for any serious condition, consult your doctor before taking this product. As with aspirin and acetaminophen, if you have any condition which requires you to take prescription drugs, or if you have had any problems or serious side effects from taking non-prescription pain relievers, do not take this product without first consulting your doctor. If you experience any symptoms which are unusual or seem unrelated to the condition for which you took this product, consult a doctor before taking any more of it. Although ibuprofen is indicated for the same conditions as aspirin and acetaminophen, it should not be taken with them except under a doctor's direction. Do not combine this product with any other ibuprofen-containing product. IT IS ESPECIALLY IMPORTANT NOT TO USE ASPIRIN DURING THE LAST 3 MONTHS OF PREGNANCY UNLESS SPECIFICALLY DIRECTED TO DO SO BY A DOCTOR BECAUSE IT MAY CAUSE PROBLEMS IN THE UNBORN CHILD OR COMPLICATIONS DURING DELIVERY.

MOTRIN IB SINUS
Pharmacia & Upjohn, Inc.

Dosage Form: caplet, tablet

Active Ingredients: pseudoephedrine hydrochloride (HCl), ibuprofen

Warning: ASPIRIN SENSITIVE PATIENTS: Do not take this product if you have had a severe allergic reaction to aspirin, e.g.—asthma, swelling, shock or hives, because even though this product contains no aspirin or salicylates, cross-reactions may occur in patients allergic to aspirin. Do not exceed recommended dosage because at higher dosages, nervousness, dizziness, or sleeplessness may occur. Do not take for colds for more than 7 days or for fever for more than 3 days

unless directed by a doctor. If the cold or fever persists or gets worse, or if new symptoms occur, consult a doctor. These could be signs of serious illness. If you are under a doctor's care for any serious condition, consult a doctor before taking this product. As with aspirin and acetaminophen, if you have any condition which requires you to take prescription drugs or if you have had any problems or serious side effects from taking any non-prescription pain reliever, do not take this product without first discussing it with your doctor. If you experience any symptoms which are unusual or seem unrelated to the condition for which you took this product, consult a doctor before taking any more of it. Do not take this product if you have heart disease, high blood pressure, thyroid disease, diabetes or difficulty in urination due to enlargement of the prostate gland, unless directed by a doctor. Do not combine this product with other non-prescription pain relievers. Do not combine this product with any other ibuprofen-containing product. DRUG INTERACTION PRECAUTION: Do not use this product if you are now taking a prescription monoamine oxidase inhibitor (MAOI) (certain drugs for depression, psychiatric or emotional conditions, or Parkinson's disease) or for 2 weeks after stopping the MAOI drug. If you are uncertain if your prescription drug contains an MAOI, consult a health professional before taking this product. IT IS ESPECIALLY IMPORTANT NOT TO USE ASPIRIN DURING THE LAST 3 MONTHS OF PREGNANCY UNLESS SPECIFICALLY DIRECTED TO DO SO BY A DOCTOR BECAUSE IT MAY CAUSE PROBLEMS IN THE UNBORN CHILD OR COMPLICATIONS DURING DELIVERY.

MURINE EARWAX REMOVAL SYSTEM
Ross Products Division, Abbott Laboratories

Dosage Form: drops

Active Ingredients: carbamide peroxide

Warning: Do not use if you have ear damage or discharge, ear pain, irritation or rash in the ear, or are dizzy; consult a doctor. Do not use if you have an injury or perforation (hole) of the eardrum or after ear surgery unless directed by a doctor. Avoid contact with the eyes. If accidental contact with eyes occurs flush eyes with water and consult a doctor. Do not use for more than 4 days. If excessive ear wax remains after use of this product, consult a doctor.

MURINE TEARS
Ross Products Division, Abbott Laboratories

Dosage Form: drops

Active Ingredients: polyvinyl alcohol, povidone

Warning: To avoid contamination do not touch tip of container to any surface. Replace cap after usage. If you experience eye pain, changes in vision, continued redness or irritation of the eye, or if the condition worsens or persists for more than 72 hours, discontinue use and consult a doctor. If the solution changes color or becomes cloudy, do not use.

MURINE TEARS PLUS
Ross Products Division, Abbott Laboratories

Dosage Form: drops

Active Ingredients: polyvinyl alcohol, povidone, tetrahydrozoline hydrochloride

Warning: To avoid contamination do not touch tip of container to any surface. Replace cap after usage. If you experience eye pain, changes in vision, continued redness or irritation of the eye, or if the condition worsens or persists for more than 72 hours, discontinue use and consult a doctor. If you have glaucoma, do not use this product except under the advice and supervision of a doctor. Overuse of this product may produce increased redness of the eye. If the solution changes color or becomes cloudy, do not use.

MYCELEX-7
Bayer Corporation, Consumer Care Division

Dosage Form: cream

Active Ingredient: clotrimazole

Warning: If this is the first time you have had vaginal itch and discomfort, consult your doctor. If you have had a doctor diagnose a vaginal yeast infection before and have the same symptoms now, use this cream as directed for 7 consecutive days. Do not use if you have abdominal pain, fever, or foul-smelling discharge. Contact your doctor immediately. If your symptoms do not improve in 3 days, or if your infection is not gone in 7 days, you may have a condition other than a yeast infection. Consult your doctor. If your symptoms return within 2 months or if you have infections that do not clear up easily with proper treatment, consult your doctor. You could be pregnant or there could be a serious underlying medical cause for your infections, including diabetes, or a damaged immune system (including damage from infection with HIV—the virus that causes AIDS). Do not rely on condoms or diaphragms to prevent sexually transmitted diseases or pregnancy while using Mycelex–7 vaginal cream. Do not use tampons while using this medication. Do not use in girls less that 12 years of age.

MYCELEX OTC ANTIFUNGAL
Bayer Corporation, Consumer Care Division

Dosage Form: cream, liquid solution

Active Ingredient: clotrimazole

Warning: For external use only. Do not use on children under 2 years of age except under the advice and supervision of a doctor. If irritation occurs or if there is no improvement within 4 weeks (for athlete's foot or ringworm) or within 2 weeks (for jock itch), discontinue use and consult a doctor or pharmacist.

MYLANTA MAXIMUM STRENGTH FAST ACTING ANTACID/ANTI-GAS
Johnson & Johnson·Merck

Dosage Form: suspension

Active Ingredients: aluminum hydroxide, magnesium hydroxide, simethicone

Warning: Do not take more than 12 teaspoonfuls in a 24 hour period, or use the maximum dosage of this product for more than 2 weeks. Do not use this product if you have kidney disease, except under the advice and supervision of a doctor. DRUG INTERACTION PRECAUTION: Antacids may interact with certain prescription drugs. If you are presently taking a prescription drug, do not take this product without checking with your physician or other health professional.

MYLANTA GAS RELIEF
Johnson & Johnson·Merck

Dosage Form: gelcap, chewable tablet

Active Ingredient: simethicone

Warning: If symptoms persist, contact your doctor.

MYOFLEX
EXTERNAL ANALGESIC CREME
Ciba Self-Medication, Inc. *

Dosage Form: cream

Active Ingredient: trolamine salicylate

Warning: For external use only. Use only as directed. Avoid contact with eyes and mucous membranes. If skin redness or irritation develops, if condition worsens, or does not improve within 7 days, or clears up and occurs again within a few days, discontinue use and consult a doctor. Do not apply to wounds, or to damaged, broken (open) or irritated skin.

NALDECON DX ADULT LIQUID
Apothecon, Division of Bristol-Myers Squibb Company

Dosage Form: liquid

Active Ingredients: phenylpropanolamine hydrochloride (HCl), guaifenesin, dextromethorphan hydrobromide

Warning: Do not give this product to children under 12 years of age unless directed by a doctor. Do not exceed recommended dosage because at higher dosages, nervousness, dizziness, or sleeplessness may occur. Do not take this product for more than 7 days. If symptoms do not improve or are accompanied by a fever, consult a doctor. Do not take this product if you have heart disease, high blood pressure, thyroid disease, diabetes or difficulty in urination due to enlargement of the prostate gland, unless directed by a doctor. A persistent cough may be a sign of a serious condition. If cough persists for more than 1 week, tends to recur, or is accompanied by a fever, rash or persistent headache, consult a doctor. Do not take this product for persistent or chronic cough such as occurs with smoking, asthma, chronic bronchitis or emphysema or when cough is accompanied by excessive phlegm (mucous) unless directed by a

doctor. May cause excitability especially in children. DRUG INTERACTION PRECAUTION: Do not use this product if you are now taking a prescription monoamine oxidase inhibitor (MAOI) (certain drugs for depression, psychiatric or emotional conditions, or Parkinson's disease) or for 2 weeks after stopping the MAOI drug. If you are uncertain if your prescription drug contains an MAOI, consult a health professional before taking this product.

NALDECON DX CHILDREN'S SYRUP
Apothecon, Division of Bristol-Myers Squibb Company

Dosage Form: syrup

Active Ingredients: phenylpropanolamine hydrochloride (HCl), guaifenesin, dextromethorphan hydrobromide

Warning: Do not exceed recommended dosage because at higher doses nervousness, dizziness, or sleeplessness may occur. Do not give this product to children for more than 7 days. If symptoms do not improve or are accompanied by a fever, consult a doctor. Do not take this product to children who have heart disease, high blood pressure, thyroid disease, or diabetes unless directed by a doctor. A persistent cough may be a sign of a serious condition. If cough persists for more than 1 week, tends to recur, or is accompanied by a fever, rash or persistent headache, consult a doctor. Do not take this product for persistent or chronic cough such as occurs with asthma, or if cough is accompanied by excessive phlegm (mucous) unless directed by a doctor. DRUG INTERACTION PRECAUTION: Do not use this product if you are now taking a prescription monoamine oxidase inhibitor (MAOI) (certain drugs for depression, psychiatric or emotional conditions, or Parkinson's disease) or for 2 weeks after stopping the MAOI drug. If you are uncertain if your prescription drug contains an MAOI, consult a health professional before taking this product.

NASAL SALINE MOISTURIZER
Bayer Corporation, Consumer Care Division

Dosage Form: drops, spray

Active Ingredients: sodium chloride

Warning: The use of this container by more than one person may spread infection.

NATURE'S REMEDY
Block Drug

Dosage Form: tablet

Active Ingredients: cascara sagrada, aloe

Warning: Do not use laxative products when abdominal pain, nausea, or vomiting are present unless directed by a doctor. If you have noticed a sudden change in bowel habits that persists over a period of 2 weeks, consult a doctor before using a laxative. Laxative products should not be used for a period longer than 1 week unless directed by a doctor. Rectal bleeding or failure to have a bowel movement after use of a laxative may indicate a serious condition. Discontinue use and consult a doctor.

NAUZENE
Alva-Amco Pharmacal

Dosage Form: tablet

Active Ingredient: diphenhydramine hydrochloride (HCl)

Warning: Do not give to children under 2 years of age unless directed by a doctor. Do not take this product, unless directed by a doctor, if you have breathing problems such as emphysema, or chronic bronchitis, or if you have glaucoma, or difficulty in urination due to enlargement of the prostate gland. May cause marked drowsiness: alcohol, sedatives, and tranquilizers may increase its drowsiness effect. Avoid alcoholic beverages while taking this product. Do not take this product if you are taking sedatives or tranquilizers, without first consulting your doctor. Use caution when driving a motor vehicle or operating machinery. Not for frequent or prolonged use, except on advice of a doctor. Do not exceed recommended dosage.

NEOSPORIN ORIGINAL
Warner Wellcome Consumer

Dosage Form: ointment

Active Ingredients: polymyxin B sulfate, bacitracin zinc, neomycin

Warning: For external use only. Do not use in the eyes or apply over large areas of the body. In case of deep or puncture wounds, animal bites or serious burns, consult a doctor. If the condition persists or gets worse, or if a rash or other allergic reaction occurs, discontinue use and consult a doctor. Do not use longer than 1 week unless directed by a doctor. Do not use this product if you are allergic to any of the listed ingredients

NEOSPORIN PLUS
MAXIMUM STRENGTH
Warner Wellcome Consumer

Dosage Form: ointment, cream

Active Ingredients: polymyxin B sulfate, bacitracin zinc, neomycin, pramoxine hydrochloride (HCl)

Warning: For external use only. Do not use in the eyes or apply over large areas of the body. In case of deep or puncture wounds, animal bites, or serious burns, consult a doctor. If the condition worsens, or if symptoms persist for more than 1 week or clear up and occur again within a few days, or if a rash or other allergic reaction develops, discontinue use of this product and consult a doctor. Do not use longer than 1 week unless directed by a doctor. Do not use in large quantities, particularly over raw surfaces or blistered areas. Do not use this product if you are allergic to any of the listed ingredients.

NERVINE NIGHTTIME SLEEP-AID
Bayer Corporation, Consumer Care Division

Dosage Form: caplet

Active Ingredient: diphenhydramine hydrochloride

Warning: Do not give to children under 12 years of age. If sleeplessness persists continuously for more than 2 weeks, consult a doctor. Insomnia may be a symptom of serious underlying medical illness. Do not take this product unless directed by a doctor, if you have breathing problems such as emphysema or chronic bronchitis, or if you have glaucoma, or difficulty in urination due to enlargement of the prostate gland. Avoid alcoholic beverages while taking this product. Do not take this product if you are taking sedatives or tranquilizers without first consulting your doctor.

NEUTROGENA CLEAR PORE TREATMENT
Neutrogena Dermatologics

Dosage Form: gel

Active Ingredient: salicylic acid

Warning: For external use only. Avoid contact with eyes. If contact occurs, flush thoroughly with water. Using other topical acne medications at the same time, or immediately following use of this product, may increase dryness or irritation of the skin. If this occurs, only one medication should be used unless directed by a doctor.

NEUTROGENA EMULSION
Neutrogena Dermatologics

Dosage Form: lotion

Active Ingredient: No active ingredients have been indicated by the manufacturer.

Warning: No warnings have been indicated by the manufacturer.

NEUTROGENA OIL-FREE ACNE WASH
Neutrogena Dermatologics

Dosage Form: liqui-gel

Active Ingredient: salicylic acid

Warning: For external use only. Avoid contact with eyes. If contact occurs, flush thoroughly with water. Using other topical acne medications at the same time or immediately following use of this product may increase dryness or irritation of the skin. If this occurs, only one medication should be used unless directed by a doctor.

NEUTROGENA THERAPEUTIC T/GEL SHAMPOO
Neutrogena Dermatologics

Dosage Form: shampoo, conditioner

Active Ingredient: coal tar

Warning: For external use only. Avoid contact with the eyes. If contact occurs, rinse eyes thoroughly with water. If condition worsens or does not improve after regular use of this product as directed, consult a doctor. Use caution in exposing skin to sunlight after applying this product. It may increase tendency to sunburn for up to 24 hours after application. Do not use for prolonged periods without consulting a doctor. Do not use this product with other forms of psoriasis therapy, such as ultraviolet radiation or prescription drugs, unless directed by a doctor. If condition covers large area of the body, consult your doctor before using this product. In rare instances, discoloration of gray, blond, bleached or tinted hair may occur.

NIVEA CREME ULTRA MOISTURIZING
Beiersdorf, Inc.

Dosage Form: cream

Active Ingredient: No active ingredients have been indicated by the manufacturer.

Warning: No warnings have been indicated by the manufacturer.

NIX LICE TREATMENT
Warner Wellcome Consumer

Dosage Form: cream rinse

Active Ingredient: permethrin

Warning: For external use only. Itching, redness, or swelling of the scalp may occur. If skin irritation persists or infection is present or develops, discontinue use and consult a doctor. Do not use near the eyes or permit contact with mucous membranes. If product gets into the eyes, immediately flush with water. Consult a doctor if infestation of eyebrows or eyelashes occurs. This product may cause breathing difficulty or an asthmatic episode in susceptible persons. This product should not be used on children less than 2 months of age.

NOLAHIST
Carnrick Laboratories, Inc.

Dosage Form: tablet

Active Ingredient: phenindamine tartrate

Warning: May cause excitability especially in children. Do not take this product if you have breathing problems such as emphysema or chronic bronchitis, or if you have glaucoma, or difficulty in urination due to enlargement of the prostate gland unless directed by a doctor. May cause drowsiness; alcohol, sedatives, and tranquilizers may increase its drowsiness effect. Avoid alcoholic beverages while taking this product. Do not take this product while taking sedatives or tranquilizers without first consulting your doctor. Use caution while driving a motor vehicle or operating machinery.

NOVAHISTINE DMX
SmithKline Beecham Consumer Health Care, L.P.

Dosage Form: syrup

Active Ingredients: pseudoephedrine hydrochloride (HCl), guaifenesin, dextromethorphan hydrobromide

Warning: Do not exceed recommended dosage because at higher dosages, nervousness, dizziness, or sleeplessness may occur. If symptoms do not improve within 7 days or are accompanied by a fever, consult a doctor. Do not take this product if you have heart disease, high blood pressure, thyroid disease, diabetes, or difficulty in urination due to enlargement of the prostate gland unless directed by a doctor. A persistent cough may be a sign of a serious condition. If cough persists for more than 1 week, tends to recur, or is accompanied by a fever, rash or persistent headache, consult a doctor. Do not take this product for persistent or chronic cough such as occurs with smoking, asthma, chronic bronchitis, or emphysema, or where cough is accompanied by excessive phlegm (mucous) unless directed by a doctor. DRUG INTERACTION PRECAUTION: Do not use this product if you are now taking a prescription monoamine oxidase inhibitor (MAOI) (certain drugs for depression, psychiatric or emotional conditions, or Parkinson's disease) or for 2 weeks after stopping the MAOI drug. If you are uncertain if your prescription drug contains an MAOI, consult a health professional before taking this product.

NUMZ-IT GEL TEETHING PAIN MEDICINE
Goody's Pharmaceuticals, Inc.

Dosage Form: gel, lotion

Active Ingredient: benzocaine

Warning: Do not use this product for more than 7 days unless directed by a dentist or doctor. If sore mouth symptoms do not improve within 7 days; if irritation, pain or redness, persists or worsens; or if swelling, rash or fever develops, see your dentist or doctor promptly. Do not exceed recommended dosage. Do not use this product if there is a history of allergy to local anesthetic products such as procaine, butacaine, benzocaine, or other "caine" anesthetics. Fever and nasal congestion are not symptoms of teething and may indicate the presence of infection. If these symptoms persist, consult a doctor. Avoid contact with the eyes.

NUPRIN PAIN RELIEF FORMULA
Bristol-Myers Products

Dosage Form: caplet, tablet

Active Ingredient: ibuprofen

Warning: ASPIRIN SENSITIVE PATIENTS: Do not take this product if you have had a severe allergic reaction to aspirin, e.g.—asthma, swelling, shock or hives, because even though this product contains no aspirin or salicylates, cross-reactions may occur in patients allergic to aspirin. Do not take this product for pain for more than 10 days or for fever for more than 3 days unless directed by a doctor. If pain or fever persists or gets worse, if new symptoms occur, or if redness or swelling is present, consult a doctor. These could be signs of serious illness. If you are under a doctor's care for any serious condition, consult your doctor before taking this product. As with aspirin and acetaminophen, if you have any condition which requires you to take prescription drugs, or if you have had any problems or serious side effects from taking non-prescription pain relievers, do not take this product without first consulting your doctor. If you experience any symptoms which are unusual or seem unrelated to the condition for which you took this product, consult a doctor before taking any more of it. Although ibuprofen is indicated for the same conditions as aspirin and acetaminophen, it should not be taken with them except under a doctor's direction. Do not combine this product with any other ibuprofen-containing product. IT IS ESPECIALLY IMPORTANT NOT TO USE ASPIRIN DURING THE LAST 3 MONTHS OF PREGNANCY UNLESS SPECIFICALLY DIRECTED TO DO SO BY A DOCTOR BECAUSE IT MAY CAUSE PROBLEMS IN THE UNBORN CHILD OR COMPLICATIONS DURING DELIVERY.

NYTOL QUICK CAPS
Block Drug

Dosage Form: caplet

Active Ingredient: diphenhydramine hydrochloride (HCl)

Warning: Do not give to children under 12 years of age. If sleeplessness persists continually for more than 2 weeks, consult a doctor. Insomnia may be a symptom of serious underlying medical illness. Do not take this product unless directed by a doctor, if you have breathing problems such as emphysema or chronic bronchitis, or if you have glaucoma, or difficulty in urination due to enlargement of the prostate gland. Avoid alcoholic beverages while taking this product. Do not take this product if you are taking sedatives or tranquilizers without first consulting your doctor.

NYTOL MAXIMUM STRENGTH NIGHTTIME SLEEP-AID
Block Drug

Dosage Form: caplet

Active Ingredient: doxylamine succinate

Warning: Do not give to children under 12 years of age. If sleeplessness persists continuously for more than 2 weeks, consult a doctor. Insomnia may be a symptom of serious underlying medical illness. Do not take this product unless directed by a doctor, if you have breathing problems such as emphysema or chronic bronchitis, or if you have glaucoma, or difficulty in urination due to enlargement of the prostate gland. Avoid alcoholic beverages while taking this product. Do not take this product while taking any other drug, without consulting your doctor or pharmacist. This product contains an antihistamine and will cause drowsiness. It should be used only at bedtime.

OCEAN
Fleming & Company

Dosage Form: spray

Active Ingredients: sodium chloride

Warning: The use of this container by more than one person may spread infection. Do not use if seal is broken or missing.

OCUCLEAR EYE REDNESS RELIEVER
Schering-Plough HealthCare Products

Dosage Form: drops

Active Ingredients: oxymetazoline hydrochloride (HCl)

Warning: To avoid contamination of this product, do not touch tip of container to any surface. Replace cap after usage. If you experience eye pain, changes in vision, continued redness or irritation of the eye, or if the condition worsens or persists for more than 72 hours, discontinue use and consult a doctor. If you have glaucoma do not use this product except under the advice and supervision of a doctor. Overuse of this product may produce increased redness of the eye. If the solution changes color or becomes cloudy, do not use. Remove soft contact lenses before using this product.

OCUREST TEARS FORMULA LUBRICANT
Occurest Laboratories

Dosage Form: drops

Active Ingredient: hydroxypropyl methylcellulose

Warning: To avoid contamination, do not touch tip of of the dispenser to any surface. Replace cap after using. If you experience eye pain, changes in vision, continued redness or irritation of the eye, or if the condition worsens or persists for more than 72 hours, discontinue use and consult a doctor. If the solution changes color or becomes cloudy, do not use. Remove contact lenses before using this product.

OFF-EZY CORN AND CALLUS REMOVER KIT
Del Pharmaceuticals, Inc.

Dosage Form: liquid

Active Ingredient: salicylic acid

Warning: For external use only. Do not use this product on irritated skin, on any area that is infected or reddened, if you are a diabetic, or if you have poor blood circulation. If discomfort persists, see your doctor. If product gets in the eyes, flush with water for 15 minutes. Avoid inhaling vapors. Flammable. Keep away from fire or flame. Cap bottle tightly and store at room temperature away from heat.

ORABASE-B WITH BENZOCAINE
Colgate-Palmolive Company

Dosage Form: paste

Active Ingredient: benzocaine

Warning: Do not use this product for more than 7 days unless directed by a dentist or doctor. If sore mouth symptoms do not improve; if irritation, pain, or redness, persists or worsens; or if swelling, rash or fever develops, discontinue use of this product and see your dentist or doctor promptly. Do not exceed recommended dosage. Do not use this product if you have a history of allergy to local anesthetics such as procaine, butacaine, benzocaine, or other "caine" anesthetics. Avoid contact with the eyes.

ORABASE BABY
Colgate-Palmolive Company

Dosage Form: gel

Active Ingredient: benzocaine

Warning: Do not use in eyes. Do not use this product for more than 7 days unless directed by a dentist or doctor. If sore mouth symptoms do not improve within 7 days, if irritation, pain or redness persists or worsens; or if swelling, rash or fever develops, see your doctor or dentist promptly. Do not exceed recommended dosage. Localized allergic reactions may occur after prolonged or repeated use. Do not use this product if there is a history of allergy to local anesthetic products such as procaine, butacaine, benzocaine, or other "caine" anesthetics.

ORABASE GEL ORAL ANALGESIC PROTECTIVE GEL
Colgate-Palmolive Company

Dosage Form: gel

Active Ingredient: benzocaine

Warning: Do not use on eyes. A mild or temporary burning sensation may be experienced upon application. If sore mouth symptoms do not improve within 7 days; or if irritation, pain or redness persists or worsens, or if swelling, rash or fever develops, discontinue use of product and see your dentist or doctor promptly. Localized allergic reactions may occur after prolonged or repeated use. Do not use this product if you have a history of allergy to local anesthetics such as procaine, butacaine, benzocaine, or other "caine" anesthetics. Avoid contact with the eyes. Do not use if printed seal on flap is broken or if tube is cut prior to opening

ORABASE LIP
Colgate-Palmolive Company

Dosage Form: cream

Active Ingredients: benzocaine, allantoin

Warning: For external use only. Avoid contact with eyes. If condition persists, or if rash, swelling or irritation develops discontinue use of this product and consult a doctor. Localized allergic reactions may occur after prolonged or repeated use. Do not use this product if you have a history of allergy to local anesthetics such as procaine, butacaine, benzocaine, or other "caine" anesthetics. Avoid contact with the eyes. As with all personal care items, this product should be used by one individual only.

ORAJEL BABY
Del Pharmaceuticals, Inc.

Dosage Form: gel

Active Ingredient: benzocaine

Warning: Do not use this product for more than 7 days unless directed by a dentist or doctor. If sore mouth symptoms do not improve within 7 days; if irritation, pain or redness, persists or worsens; or if swelling, rash or fever develops, see your doctor or dentist promptly. Do not exceed recommended dosage. Do not use this product if you have a history of allergy to local anesthetics such as procaine, butacaine, benzocaine, or other "caine" anesthetics. Fever and nasal congestion are not symptoms of teething and may indicate the presence of infection. If these symptoms persist, consult your doctor. Avoid contact with the eyes.

ORAJEL MAXIMUM STRENGTH
Del Pharmaceuticals, Inc.

Dosage Form: gel

Active Ingredient: benzocaine

Warning: Do not use if tube tip is cut prior to opening. Do not use this product if you have a history of allergy to local anesthetics such as procaine, butacaine, benzocaine, or other "caine" anesthetics.

ORAJEL MOUTH-AID
Del Pharmaceuticals, Inc.

Dosage Form: gel

Active Ingredients: benzocaine, zinc chloride

Warning: Do not use this product for more than 7 days unless directed by a dentist or doctor. If sore mouth symptoms do not improve; if irritation, pain, or redness, persists or worsens; or if swelling, rash or fever develops, discontinue use of this product and see your dentist or doctor promptly. Do not exceed recommended dosage. Do not use this product if you have a history of allergy to local anesthetics such as procaine, butacaine, benzocaine, or other "caine" anesthetics. Avoid contact with the eyes.

ORUDIS KT
Whitehall-Robins Healthcare

Dosage Form: caplet, tablet

Active Ingredient: ketoprofen

Warning: Do not take this product if you have had asthma, hives or any other severe allergic reaction after taking any pain reliever/fever reducer. Ketoprofen could cause similar reactions in patients allergic to other pain relievers/fever reducers. If you generally consume 3 or more alcohol-containing drinks per day you should talk to you doctor for advice on when and how you should take Orudis KT or other pain relievers. Do not use: with any other pain reliever/fever reducers; with any other product containing Ketoprofen; for more than 3 days for fever; for more than 10 days for pain. Ask a doctor before use if: the painful area is red or swollen; you take regular drugs on a regular basis; you are under a doctor's care for any continuing medical condition; you have had problems or side effects with any pain reliever/fever reducers. Ask a doctor after use if: symptoms continue or worsen; new or unexpected symptoms occur; stomach pains occur with use of product. IT IS ESPECIALLY IMPORTANT NOT TO USE ASPIRIN DURING THE LAST 3 MONTHS OF PREGNANCY UNLESS SPECIFICALLY DIRECTED TO DO SO BY A DOCTOR BECAUSE IT MAY CAUSE PROBLEMS IN THE UNBORN CHILD OR COMPLICATIONS DURING DELIVERY.

OXY 10 DAILY FACE ACNE WASH
SmithKline Beecham
Consumer Health Care, L.P.

Dosage Form: liquid

Active Ingredient: benzoyl peroxide

Warning: For external use only. Keep away from eyes, lips, mouth and sensitive areas of the neck. If contact with eyes occurs, flush thoroughly with water. Using other topical acne medications at the same time or immediately following use of this product may increase dryness or irritation of the skin. If this occurs, only one medication should be used unless directed by a doctor. Do not use this medication if you have very sensitive skin or are sensitive to benzoyl peroxide. This product may cause irritation, characterized by redness, burning, itching, peeling or possibly swelling. More frequent use or higher concentrations may aggravate such irritation. Mild irritation may be reduced by using the product less frequently or in a lower concentration. If irritation becomes severe, discontinue

use; if irritation still continues consult your doctor. This product may bleach hair or dyed fabrics.

OXY 10 MAXIMUM STRENGTH ACNE TREATMENT
SmithKline Beecham
Consumer Health Care, L.P.

Dosage Form: lotion

Active Ingredient: benzoyl peroxide

Warning: For external use only. Keep away from eyes, lips, mouth and sensitive areas of the neck. If contact with eyes occurs, flush thoroughly with water. Using other topical acne medications at the same time or immediately following use of this product may increase dryness or irritation of the skin. If this occurs, only one medication should be used unless directed by a doctor. Do not use this medication if you have very sensitive skin or if you are sensitive to benzoyl peroxide. This product may cause irritation, characterized by redness, burning, itching, peeling, or possibly swelling. More frequent use or higher concentrations may aggravate such irritation. Mild irritation may be reduced by using the product less frequently or in a lower concentration. If irritation becomes severe, discontinue use; if irritation still continues, consult a doctor. This product may bleach hair or dyed fabrics.

P

PACQUIN MEDICATED HAND & BODY
Pfizer Inc., Consumer Care Group

Dosage Form: cream

Warning: No warnings have been indicated by the manufacturer.

PANADOL CHILDREN'S
Bayer Corporation,
Consumer Care Division

Dosage Form: liquid, chewable tablet

Active Ingredient: acetaminophen

Warning: Do not take this product for pain for more than 5 days or for fever for more than 3 days unless directed by a doctor. If pain or fever persists or gets worse, if new symptoms occur, or if redness or swelling is present, consult a doctor. These could be signs of serious illness. Do not use with other products containing acetaminophen.

PAREPECTOLIN
Rhône-Poulenc Rorer
Pharmaceuticals, Inc.

Dosage Form: suspension

Active Ingredient: attapulgite

Warning: Do not use for more than 2 days unless directed by a doctor. Do not use if diarrhea is accompanied by a fever,

or if blood or mucus is present in the stool. Do not use in infants or children under 3 years of age unless directed by a doctor. If you are taking a prescription medicine, consult your doctor before taking this product.

PEDIACARE INFANTS' DECONGESTANT DROPS
McNeil Consumer Products Company

Dosage Form: drops

Active Ingredient: pseudoephedrine hydrochloride (HCl)

Warning: If nervousness, dizziness, or sleeplessness occur, discontinue use and consult a doctor. If symptoms do not improve within 7 days or are accompanied by a fever, consult a doctor. Do not give this product to a child who has heart disease, high blood pressure, diabetes or thyroid disease unless directed by a doctor. DRUG INTERACTION PRECAUTION: Do not use this product if you are now taking a prescription monoamine oxidase inhibitor (MAOI) (certain drugs for depression, psychiatric or emotional conditions, or Parkinson's disease) or for 2 weeks after stopping the MAOI drug. If you are uncertain if your prescription drug contains an MAOI, consult a health professional before taking this product

PEDIACARE NIGHTREST COUGH-COLD
McNeil Consumer Products Company

Dosage Form: liquid

Active Ingredients: pseudoephedrine hydrochloride (HCl), chlorpheniramine maleate, dextromethorphan hydrobromide

Warning: Do not exceed recommended dosage because at higher dosages, nervousness, dizziness, or sleeplessness may occur. If symptoms do not improve within 7 days or are accompanied by a fever, consult a doctor. A persistent cough may be a sign of a serious condition. If cough persists for more than 1 week, tends to recur, or is accompanied by a fever, rash or persistent headache, consult a doctor. Do not take this product for persistent or chronic cough such as occurs with asthma, chronic bronchitis, or emphysema, or if cough is accompanied by excessive phlegm (mucous) unless directed by a doctor. May cause excitability especially in children. May cause drowsiness; sedatives, and tranquilizers may increase its drowsiness effect. Do not give this product to children who are taking sedatives or tranquilizers without first consulting the child's doctor. Do not give this product to children who have a breathing problem such as chronic bronchitis, heart disease, high blood pressure, thyroid disease, diabetes or glaucoma without first consulting a doctor. DRUG INTERACTION PRECAUTION: Do not use this product if you are now taking a prescription monoamine oxidase inhibitor (MAOI) (certain drugs for depression, psychiatric or emotional conditions, or Parkinson's disease) or for 2 weeks after stopping the MAOI drug. If you are uncertain if your prescription drug contains an MAOI, consult a health professional before taking this product.

PEPCID AC ACID CONTROLLER
Johnson & Johnson·Merck

Dosage Form: tablet

Active Ingredient: famotidine

Warning: Do not take the maximum daily dosage for more than 2 weeks continuously, except under the advice and supervision of a doctor. CAUTION: Heartburn and acid indigestion are common, but you should see your doctor promptly if you have used the maximum dosage every day for 2 weeks continuously, or if you have trouble swallowing, or persistent abdominal pain. You may have a serious condition that may need different treatment.

PEPTO-BISMOL MAXIMUM STRENGTH
The Procter & Gamble Company

Dosage Form: liquid

Active Ingredient: bismuth subsalicylate

Warning: Children and teenagers who have or are recovering from chicken pox or flu should not use this medicine to treat nausea or vomiting. If nausea or vomiting is present, consult a doctor because this could be an early sign of Reye Syndrome, a rare but serious illness. This product contains salicylates. If taken with aspirin and ringing in the ears occurs, stop using. This product does not contain aspirin, but if you are allergic to aspirin do not use as an adverse reaction may occur. DRUG INTERACTION PRECAUTION: If you are taking medicines for anticoagulation (thinning of the blood), diabetes or gout, consult a doctor before taking this product. If diarrhea is accompanied by a high fever or continues more than 2 days, consult a doctor.

PERDIEM FIBER
Ciba Self-Medication, Inc.

Dosage Form: granule

Active Ingredients: psyllium

Warning: Persons with esophageal narrowing should not use bulk-forming agents. Do not use this product when abdominal pain, nausea or vomiting are present unless directed by a doctor. If you have noticed a sudden change in bowel habits that persists over a period of 2 weeks, consult a doctor before using a laxative. Laxative products should not be used for a period longer than 1 week unless directed by a doctor. Rectal bleeding or failure to have a bowel movement after use of a laxative may indicate a serious condition. Discontinue use and consult a doctor. Do not use if you have a history of psyllium allergy. TAKING THIS PRODUCT WITHOUT ADEQUATE FLUID MAY CAUSE IT TO SWELL AND BLOCK YOUR THROAT OR ESOPHAGUS AND MAY CAUSE CHOKING. DO NOT TAKE THIS PRODUCT IF YOU HAVE DIFFICULTY IN SWALLOWING. IF YOU EXPERIENCE CHEST PAIN, VOMITING, OR DIFFICULTY IN SWALLOWING OR BREATHING AFTER TAKING THIS PRODUCT SEEK IMMEDIATE MEDICAL ATTENTION.

PERTUSSIN DM EXTRA STRENGTH COUGH RELIEF
Blairex Laboratories, Inc.

Dosage Form: liquid

Active Ingredient: dextromethorphan hydrobromide

Warning: A persistent cough may be a sign of a serious condition. If cough persists for more than 1 week, tends to recur, or is accompanied by a fever, rash or persistent headache, consult a doctor. Do not take this product for persistent or chronic cough such as occurs with smoking, asthma, chronic bronchitis, emphysema, or where cough is accompanied by excessive phlegm (mucous) unless directed by a doctor. DRUG INTERACTION PRECAUTION: Do not use this product if you are now taking a prescription monoamine oxidase inhibitor (MAOI) (certain drugs for depression, psychiatric or emotional conditions, or Parkinson's disease) or for 2 weeks after stopping the MAOI drug. If you are uncertain if your prescription drug contains an MAOI, consult a health professional before taking this product.

PHAZYME GAS RELIEF (95MG)
Block Drug

Dosage Form: tablet

Active Ingredient: simethicone

Warning: If conditions persist, consult your doctor.

PHILIP'S MILK OF MAGNESIA LAXATIVE/ANTACID
Schein Ph'cal

Dosage Form: suspension

Active Ingredient: magnesium hydroxide

Warning: LAXATIVE WARNINGS: Do not use laxative products when abdominal pain, nausea, vomiting, or kidney disease are present unless directed by a doctor. If you have noticed a sudden change in bowel habits that persists over a period of 2 weeks, consult a doctor before using a laxative. Laxative products should not be used for a period longer than 1 week unless directed by a doctor. Rectal bleeding or failure to have a bowel movement after use of a laxative may indicate a serious condition. Discontinue use and consult a doctor. ANTACID WARNINGS: Do not take more than the maximum recommended daily dosage in a 24 hour period (see directions), or use the maximum dosage of this product for more than 2 weeks, or use this product if you have kidney disease, except under the advice and supervision of a doctor. May have laxative effect. DRUG INTERACTION PRECAUTION: Antacids may interact with certain prescription drugs. If you are presently taking a prescription drug, do not take this product without checking with your doctor or other health professional.

PHISODERM DAILY SKIN CLEANSER & CONDITIONER
Chattem, Inc.

Dosage Form: cream

Active Ingredient: No active ingredients have been indicated by the manufacturer.

Warning: No warnings have been indicated by the manufacturer.

POLYSPORIN FIRST AID ANTIBIOTIC
Warner Wellcome Consumer

Dosage Form: ointment

Active Ingredients: polymyxin B sulfate, bacitracin zinc

Warning: For external use only. Do not use in the eyes or apply over large areas of the body. In case of deep or puncture wounds, animal bites or serious burns, consult a doctor. If the condition persists or gets worse, or if a rash or other allergic reaction occurs, discontinue use and consult a doctor. Do not use longer than 1 week unless directed by a doctor. Do not use this product if you are allergic to any of the listed ingredients.

PREPARATION H
Whitehall-Robins Healthcare

Dosage Form: ointment, cream

Active Ingredient: phenylephrine hydrochloride (HCl)

Warning: If condition worsens or pain persists for more than 7 days, or clears up and occurs again within a few days, discontinue use and consult a doctor. Do not exceed the recommended daily dosage unless directed by a doctor. In case of bleeding, consult a doctor promptly. Do not use this product with an applicator. If the introduction of the applicator into the rectum causes additional pain, consult a doctor promptly. Do not use this product if you have heart disease, high blood pressure, thyroid disease, diabetes, or difficulty in urination due to the enlargement of the prostate gland unless directed by a doctor. DRUG INTERACTION PRECAUTION: Do not use this product if you are presently taking a prescription drug for high blood pressure or depression, without first consulting your doctor.

PRONTO LICE KILLING SHAMPOO
Del Pharmaceuticals, Inc.

Dosage Form: shampoo

Active Ingredients: piperonyl butoxide, pyrethrins

Warning: Use with caution on persons allergic to ragweed. For external use only. Do not use near the eyes or permit contact with mucous membranes such as inside the nose, mouth, or vagina, as irritation may occur. Keep out of eyes when rinsing hair. *Adults and children:* Close eyes tightly and do not open eyes until product is rinsed out. Also, protect children's eyes with washcloth, towel or other suitable material, or by similar method. If product gets into the eyes, immediately flush with water. If skin irritation or infection is present or develops, discontinue use and consult a doctor. Consult a doctor if infestation of eyebrows or eyelashes occurs. Wash thoroughly with soap and water after handling. Do not exceed two applications within a 24 hour period.

PROPA PH FOAMING FACE WASH
Del Pharmaceuticals, Inc.

Dosage Form: liquid

Active Ingredient: salicylic acid

Warning: For external use only. Avoid contact with eyes. If contact occurs, flush thoroughly with water. Using other topical acne medications at the same time or immediately following use of this product may increase dryness or irritation of the skin. If this occurs, only one medication should be used unless directed by a doctor.

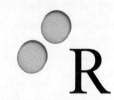

RED CROSS TOOTHACHE MEDICATION
Mentholatum Company, Inc.

Dosage Form: drops

Active Ingredient: eugenol

Warning: Do not swallow. Do not use this product for more than 7 days. If irritation persists, inflammation develops, or if fever or infection develop, discontinue use and see your dentist or doctor promptly. Do not exceed recommended dosage. Do not use if you are allergic to Eugenol. Children under 2 years should not use this product. Children under 12 years should be supervised in the use of this product.

REFRESH
Allergan, Inc.

Dosage Form: drops

Active Ingredients: polyvinyl alcohol, povidone

Warning: To avoid contamination, do not touch tip of container to any surface. Do not reuse. Once open, discard. If you experience eye pain, changes in vision, continued redness or irritation of the eye, or if the condition worsens or persists for more than 72 hours, discontinue use and consult a doctor. If the solution changes color or becomes cloudy, do not use.

REPLENS
Warner Wellcome Consumer

Dosage Form: gel

Active Ingredients: No active ingredients have been indicated by the manufacturer.

Warning: Is not a contraceptive.

RHULI GEL
Rydelle Laboratories

Dosage Form: gel

Active Ingredients: menthol, camphor

Warning: For external use only. Avoid contact with eyes. If condition does not improve or recurs within 7 days, discontinue use and consult a doctor.

RHULI SPRAY
Rydelle Laboratories

Dosage Form: spray

Active Ingredients: calamine, benzocaine, camphor

Warning: For external use only. Avoid contact with eyes. If condition does not improve or recurs within 7 days, discontinue use and consult a doctor.

RICOLA
Ricola USA, Inc.

Dosage Form: lozenge

Active Ingredient: menthol

Warning: If sore throat is severe, persists for more than 2 days, or is accompanied or followed by a fever, headache, rash, swelling, nausea or vomiting, consult a doctor promptly. If sore mouth symptoms do not improve within 7 days, or if irritation, pain, or redness persists or worsens, see your dentist or doctor promptly. Do not exceed recommended dosage. Do not administer to children under 3 years of age unless directed by a doctor. May have a laxative effect if consumed in large quantities.

RID LICE KILLING SHAMPOO MAXIMUM STRENGTH
Pfizer Inc., Consumer Care Group

Dosage Form: shampoo

Active Ingredients: piperonyl butoxide, pyrethrum

Warning: Use with caution on persons allergic to ragweed. For external use only. Do not use near the eyes or permit contact with mucous membranes such as inside the nose, mouth, or vagina, as irritation may occur. Keep out of eyes when rinsing hair. *Adults and children:* Close eyes tightly and do not open eyes until product is rinsed out. Also, protect children's eyes with washcloth, towel or other suitable material, or by similar method. If product gets into the eyes, immediately flush with water. If skin irritation or infection is present or develops, discontinue use and consult a doctor. Consult a doctor if infestation of eyebrows or eyelashes occurs.

RIOPAN PLUS DOUBLE STRENGTH ANTACID & ANTI-GAS
Whitehall-Robins Healthcare

Dosage Form: suspension

Active Ingredient: magaldrate, simethicone

Warning: Do not take more than 12 teaspoonfuls in a 24-hour period or use the maximum dosage of this product for more than 2 weeks. Do not use this product if you have kidney disease, except under the advice and supervision of a doctor. DRUG INTERACTION PRECAUTION: Antacids may interact with certain prescription drugs. If you are presently taking a prescription drug, do not take this product without checking with your doctor or other health professional.

ROBITUSSIN
Whitehall-Robins Healthcare

Dosage Form: syrup

Active Ingredient: guaifenesin

Warning: Do not take this product for persistent or chronic cough such as occurs with smoking, asthma, chronic bronchitis, emphysema, or where cough is accompanied by excessive phlegm (mucous) unless directed by a doctor. A persistent cough may be a sign of a serious condition. If cough persists for more than 1 week, tends to recur, or is accompanied by a fever, rash or persistent headache, consult a doctor. Do not take this product if you are hypersensitive to any of the ingredients. As with any drug, if you

are pregnant or nursing a baby, seek the advice of a health care professional before using this product.

ROBITUSSIN CF
Whitehall-Robins Healthcare

Dosage Form: syrup

Active Ingredients: phenylpropanolamine hydrochloride (HCl), guaifenesin, dextromethorphan hydrobromide

Warning: Do not exceed recommended dosage because at higher dosages, nervousness, dizziness, or sleeplessness may occur. Do not take this product for more than 7 days. Do not take this product if you have heart disease, high blood pressure, thyroid disease, diabetes, or difficulty in urination due to enlargement of the prostate gland unless directed by a doctor. A persistent cough may be a sign of a serious condition. If cough persists for more than 1 week, tends to recur, or is accompanied by a fever, rash or persistent headache, consult a doctor. Do not take this product for persistent or chronic cough such as occurs with smoking, asthma, chronic bronchitis, or emphysema, or where cough is accompanied by excessive phlegm (mucous) unless directed by a doctor. DRUG INTERACTION PRECAUTION: Do not use this product if you are now taking a prescription monoamine oxidase inhibitor (MAOI) (certain drugs for depression, psychiatric or emotional conditions, or Parkinson's disease) or for 2 weeks after stopping the MAOI drug. If you are uncertain if your prescription drug contains an MAOI, consult a health professional before taking this product.

ROBITUSSIN COUGH DROPS
Whitehall-Robins Healthcare

Dosage Form: lozenge

Active Ingredients: menthol

Warning: A persistent cough or sore throat may be a sign of a serious condition. If cough persists for more than 1 week, tends to recur, or is accompanied by fever, rash, or persistent headache, or a sore throat is severe, persistent or accompanied by high fever, headache, nausea and vomiting, consult a doctor. Do not take this product for a sore throat lasting more than 2 days or for a persistent or chronic cough such as occurs with smoking, asthma, emphysema or if cough is accompanied by excessive phlegm (mucous) unless directed by a doctor.

ROBITUSSIN DM
Whitehall-Robins Healthcare

Dosage Form: syrup

Active Ingredients: guaifenesin, dextromethorphan hydrobromide

Warning: A persistent cough may be a sign of a serious condition. If cough persists for more than 1 week, tends to recur, or is accompanied by a fever, rash or persistent headache, consult a doctor. Do not take this product for persistent or chronic cough such as occurs with smoking, asthma, chronic bronchitis, or emphysema, or where cough is accompanied by excessive phlegm (mucous) unless directed by a doctor. Do not take this product if you are hypersensitive to any of its ingredients. DRUG INTERACTION PRECAUTION: Do not use this product if you are now taking a prescription monoamine oxidase inhibitor (MAOI) (certain drugs for depression, psychiatric or emotional conditions, or Parkinson's disease) or for 2 weeks after stopping the MAOI drug. If you are uncertain if your prescription drug contains an MAOI, consult a health professional before taking this product.

ROBITUSSIN MAXIMUM STRENGTH COUGH
Whitehall-Robins Healthcare

Dosage Form: liquid

Active Ingredient: dextromethorphan hydrobromide

Warning: A persistent cough may be a sign of a serious condition. If cough persists for more than 1 week, tends to recur, or is accompanied by a fever, rash, or persistent headache consult a doctor. Do not take this product for persistent or chronic cough such as occurs with smoking, asthma, chronic bronchitis, emphysema, or if cough is accompanied by excessive phlegm (mucous) unless directed by a doctor. DRUG INTERACTION PRECAUTION: Do not use this product if you are now taking a prescription monoamine oxidase inhibitor (MAOI) (certain drugs for depression, psychiatric or emotional conditions, or Parkinson's disease) or for 2 weeks after stopping the MAOI drug. If you are uncertain if your prescription drug contains an MAOI, consult a health professional before taking this product.

ROBITUSSIN NIGHT-TIME COLD FORMULA
Whitehall-Robins Healthcare

Dosage Form: softgel

Active Ingredients: pseudoephedrine hydrochloride (HCl), doxylamine succinate, acetaminophen, dextromethorphan hydrobromide

Warning: Do not exceed recommended dosage. If nervousness, dizziness, or sleeplessness occur, discontinue use and consult a doctor. Do not use this product for more than 7 days. If symptoms do not improve or are accompanied by a fever that lasts for more than 3 days, or if new symptoms occur, or if redness or swelling is present, consult a doctor. These could be signs of a serious condition. If sore throat is severe, persists for more than 2 days, or is accompanied or followed by a fever, headache, rash, nausea or vomiting, consult a doctor promptly. A persistent cough may be a sign of a serious condition. If cough persists for more than 1 week, tends to recur, or is accompanied by a fever, rash or persistent headache, consult a doctor. Do not take this product for persistent or chronic cough such as occurs with asthma or if cough is accompanied by excessive phlegm (mucous) unless directed by a doctor. Do not take this product, if you have a breathing problem such as emphysema or chronic bronchitis, or if you have glaucoma, high blood pressure, heart disease, thyroid disease, diabetes or difficulty in urination due to the enlargement of the prostate gland, without first consulting a doctor. May cause excitability especially in children. May cause marked drowsiness; alcohol, sedatives, and tranquil-

izers may increase its drowsiness effect. Avoid alcoholic beverages while taking this product. Use caution while driving a motor vehicle or operating machinery. Do not use with other products containing acetaminophen. DRUG INTERACTION PRECAUTION: Do not use this product if you are now taking a prescription monoamine oxidase inhibitor (MAOI) (certain drugs for depression, psychiatric or emotional conditions, or Parkinson's disease) or for 2 weeks after stopping the MAOI drug. If you are uncertain if your prescription drug contains an MAOI, consult a health professional before taking this product.

ROBITUSSIN PEDIATRIC
Whitehall-Robins Healthcare

Dosage Form: drops

Active Ingredients: pseudoephedrine hydrochloride (HCl), guaifenesin, dextromethorphan hydrobromide

Warning: Do not exceed recommended dosage because at higher dosages, nervousness, dizziness, or sleeplessness may occur. Do not take this product for more than 7 days. If symptoms do not improve or are accompanied by a fever, consult a doctor. Do not take this product if you have heart disease, high blood pressure, thyroid disease, diabetes, or difficulty in urination due to enlargement of the prostate gland unless directed by a doctor. A persistent cough may be a sign of a serious condition. If cough persists for more than 1 week, tends to recur, or is accompanied by a fever, rash or persistent headache, consult a doctor. Do not take this product for persistent or chronic cough such as occurs with smoking, asthma, chronic bronchitis, or emphysema, or where cough is accompanied by excessive phlegm (mucous) unless directed by a doctor. DRUG INTERACTION PRECAUTION: Do not use this product if you are now taking a prescription monoamine oxidase inhibitor (MAOI) (certain drugs for depression, psychiatric or emotional conditions, or Parkinson's disease) or for 2 weeks after stopping the MAOI drug. If you are uncertain if your prescription drug contains an MAOI, consult a health professional before taking this product.

ROBITUSSIN PEDIATRIC COUGH
Whitehall-Robins Healthcare

Dosage Form: liquid

Active Ingredient: dextromethorphan hydrobromide

Warning: A persistent cough may be a sign of a serious condition. If cough persists for more than 1 week, tends to recur, or is accompanied by a fever, rash, or persistent headache consult a doctor. Do not take this product for persistent or chronic cough such as occurs with smoking, asthma, chronic bronchitis, emphysema, or if cough is accompanied by excessive phlegm (mucous) unless directed by a doctor. Do not take this product if you are hypersensitive to any of its ingredients. DRUG INTERACTION PRECAUTION: Do not use this product if you are now taking a prescription monoamine oxidase

inhibitor (MAOI) (certain drugs for depression, psychiatric or emotional conditions, or Parkinson's disease) or for 2 weeks after stopping the MAOI drug. If you are uncertain if your prescription drug contains an MAOI, consult a health professional before taking this product.

ROLAIDS ANTACID TABLETS
Warner-Lambert

Dosage Form: chewable tablet

Active Ingredients: calcium carbonate, magnesium hydroxide

Warning: Do not take more than 12 tablets in a 24-hour period or use the maximum dosage of this product for more than 2 weeks except under the advice and supervision of a doctor. DRUG INTERACTION PRECAUTION: Antacids may interact with certain prescription drugs. If you are presently taking a prescription drug, do not take this product without checking with your doctor or other health professional.

S

SEBULEX MEDICATED DANDRUFF SHAMPOO
Westwood-Squibb Pharmaceuticals

Dosage Form: shampoo

Active Ingredients: sulfur, salicylic acid

Warning: For external use only. Avoid contact with the eyes. If contact occurs, rinse eyes thoroughly with water. If undue irritation develops or increases, discontinue use and consult a doctor.

SEBUTONE TAR SHAMPOO
Westwood-Squibb Pharmaceuticals

Dosage Form: shampoo

Active Ingredient: coal tar

Warning: For external use only. Avoid contact with the eyes. If contact occurs, rinse eyes thoroughly with water. Use caution in exposing skin to sunlight after applying this product. It may increase tendency to sunburn for up to 24 hours after application. Do not use for prolonged periods without consulting a doctor. Do not use this product with other forms of psoriasis therapy, such as ultraviolet radiation or prescription drugs, unless directed by a doctor. If undo irritation develops or increases, discontinue use and consult a doctor. In rare instances, temporary discoloration of white, blond, bleached or tinted hair may occur.

SELSUN BLUE DANDRUFF SHAMPOO MEDICATED TREATMENT
Ross Products/Abbott Laboratories

Dosage Form: shampoo

Active Ingredient: selenium sulfide

Warning: For external use only. Avoid contact with the eyes. If contact occurs, rinse eyes thoroughly with water. If condition worsens or does not improve after regular use of this product as directed, consult a doctor.

SENOKOT
The Purdue Frederick Company

Dosage Form: suppository

Active Ingredient: senna concentrate

Warning: For rectal use only. Do not use laxative products when abdominal pain, nausea, or vomiting are present unless directed by a doctor. If you have noticed a sudden change in the child's bowel habits that persists over a period of 2 weeks, consult a doctor before using a laxative. Laxative products should not be used for a period longer than 1 week unless directed by a doctor. Rectal bleeding or failure to have a bowel movement after use of a laxative may indicate a serious condition. Discontinue use and consult a doctor.

SENOKOT CHILDREN'S SYRUP
The Purdue Frederick Company

Dosage Form: syrup

Active Ingredients: senna concentrate, sennosides

Warning: Do not use laxative products when abdominal pain, nausea, or vomiting are present unless directed by a doctor. If you have noticed a sudden change in the child's bowel habits that persists over a period of 2 weeks, consult a doctor before using a laxative. Laxative products should not be used for a period longer than 1 week unless directed by a doctor. Rectal bleeding or failure to have a bowel movement after use of a laxative may indicate a serious condition. Discontinue use and consult a doctor.

SENSOGARD CANKER SORE RELIEF
Dentco, Inc.

Dosage Form: gel

Active Ingredients: benzocaine, chlorpheniramine maleate

Warning: Do not use this product for more than 7 days unless directed by a dentist or doctor. If sore mouth symptoms do not improve; if irritation, pain, or redness, persists or worsens; or if swelling, rash or fever develops, discontinue use of this product and see your dentist or doctor promptly. Do not exceed recommended dosage. Do not use this product if you have a history of allergy to local anesthetics such as procaine, butacaine, benzocaine, or other "caine" anesthetics. Avoid contact with the eyes.

SINAREST EXTRA STRENGTH
Ciba Self-Medication, Inc.*

Dosage Form: tablet

Active Ingredients: pseudoephedrine hydrochloride (HCl), chlorpheniramine maleate, acetaminophen

Warning: Do not exceed recommended dosage because at higher dosages, nervousness, dizziness, or sleepiness may occur. Do not take this product for more than 10 days (for adults) or 5 days (for children). If symptoms do not improve or are accompanied by a fever that lasts for more than 3 days, or if new symptoms occur, consult a doctor. Do not take this product if you have a breathing problem such as

emphysema or chronic bronchitis, or if you have heart disease, high blood pressure, diabetes, thyroid disease, glaucoma, or difficulty in urination due to enlargement of the prostate gland unless directed by a doctor. May cause excitability especially in children. May cause drowsiness; alcohol, sedatives, and tranquilizers may increase its drowsiness effect. Avoid alcoholic beverages while taking this product. Do not take this product if you are taking sedatives or tranquilizers without first consulting your doctor. Use caution while driving a motor vehicle or operating machinery. Do not use with other products containing acetaminophen. DRUG INTERACTION PRECAUTION: Do not use this product if you are now taking a prescription monoamine oxidase inhibitor (MAOI) (certain drugs for depression, psychiatric or emotional conditions, or Parkinson's disease) or for 2 weeks after stopping the MAOI drug. If you are uncertain if your prescription drug contains an MAOI, consult a health professional before taking this product.

SINAREST NO DROWSINESS
Ciba Self-Medication, Inc.*

Dosage Form: tablet

Active Ingredients: pseudoephedrine hydrochloride (HCl), acetaminophen

Warning: Do not exceed recommended dosage because at higher dosages, nervousness, dizziness, or sleepiness may occur. Do not take this product for more than 10 days (for adults) or 5 days (for children). If symptoms do not improve or are accompanied by a fever that lasts for more than 3 days, or if new symptoms occur, consult a doctor. Do not take this product if you have heart disease, high blood pressure, thyroid disease, diabetes or difficulty in urination due to enlargement of the prostate gland, unless directed by a doctor. If you generally consume 3 or more alcohol-containing drinks per day, you should consult your doctor for advice on when and how you should take this product and other pain relievers. Do not use with other products containing acetaminophen. DRUG INTERACTION PRECAUTION: Do not use this product if you are now taking a prescription monoamine oxidase inhibitor (MAOI) (certain drugs for depression, psychiatric or emotional conditions, or Parkinson's disease) or for 2 weeks after stopping the MAOI drug. If you are uncertain if your prescription drug contains an MAOI, consult a health professional before taking this product

SINE-AID MAXIMUM STRENGTH
McNeil Consumer Products Company

Dosage Form: caplet, gelcap, tablet

Active Ingredients: pseudoephedrine hydrochloride (HCl), acetaminophen

Warning: Do not exceed recommended dosage because at higher dosages, nervousness, dizziness or sleepiness may occur. Do not take for pain for more than 7 days or for fever for more than 3 days unless directed by a doctor. If pain or fever persists, or gets worse, if new symptoms occur, or if redness or swelling is present, consult a doctor. These could be signs of serious illness. Do not take this product if you have

heart disease, high blood pressure, thyroid disease, diabetes or difficulty in urination due to enlargement of the prostate gland, unless directed by a doctor. If you generally consume 3 or more alcohol-containing drinks per day, you should consult your doctor for advice on when and how you should take this product and other pain relievers. Do not use with other products containing acetaminophen. DRUG INTERACTION PRECAUTION: Do not use this product if you are now taking a prescription monoamine oxidase inhibitor (MAOI) (certain drugs for depression, psychiatric or emotional conditions, or Parkinson's disease) or for 2 weeks after stopping the MAOI drug. If you are uncertain if your prescription drug contains an MAOI, consult a health professional before taking this product.

SINE-OFF SINUS MEDICINE
Hogil Pharmaceutical Corporation

Dosage Form: caplet

Active Ingredients: pseudoephedrine hydrochloride (HCl), chlorpheniramine maleate, acetaminophen

Warning: Do not exceed recommended dosage because at higher dosages, nervousness, dizziness, or sleepiness may occur. Do not take this product for more than 10 days. If symptoms do not improve or are accompanied by fever that lasts for more than 3 days, or if new symptoms occur, consult a doctor. Do not take this product if you have a breathing problem such as emphysema or chronic bronchitis, or if you have heart disease, high blood pressure, diabetes, thyroid disease, glaucoma or difficulty in urination due to enlargement of the prostate gland unless directed by a doctor. May cause excitability especially in children. May cause drowsiness; alcohol, sedatives, and tranquilizers may increase its drowsiness effect. Avoid alcoholic beverages while taking this product. Do not take this product if you are taking sedatives or tranquilizers without first consulting your doctor. Use caution while driving a motor vehicle or operating machinery. Do not use with other products containing acetaminophen. DRUG INTERACTION PRECAUTION: Do not use this product if you are now taking a prescription monoamine oxidase inhibitor (MAOI) (certain drugs for depression, psychiatric or emotional conditions, or Parkinson's disease) or for 2 weeks after stopping the MAOI drug. If you are uncertain if your prescription drug contains an MAOI, consult a health professional before taking this product.

SINUTAB SINUS ALLERGY MAXIMUM STRENGTH
Warner Wellcome Consumer

Dosage Form: caplet, tablet

Active Ingredients: pseudoephedrine hydrochloride (HCl), chlorpheniramine maleate, acetaminophen

Warning: Do not exceed recommended dosage because at higher dosages, nervousness, dizziness, or sleepiness may occur. Do not take this product for more than 10 days. If symptoms do not improve or are accompanied by fever that lasts for more than 3 days, or if new symptoms occur, consult a doctor. Do not take this product if you have a breathing problem such as emphysema or chronic bronchitis, or if you have heart disease, high blood pressure, diabetes, thyroid disease, glaucoma or difficulty in urination due to enlargement of the prostate gland unless directed by a doctor. May cause excitability especially in children. May cause drowsiness; alcohol, sedatives, and tranquilizers may increase its drowsiness effect. Avoid alcoholic beverages while taking this product. Do not take this product if you are taking sedatives or tranquilizers without first consulting your doctor. Use caution while driving a motor vehicle or operating machinery. Do not use with other products containing acetaminophen. DRUG INTERACTION PRECAUTION: Do not use this product if you are now taking a prescription monoamine oxidase inhibitor (MAOI) (certain drugs for depression, psychiatric or emotional conditions, or for Parkinson's disease) or for 2 weeks after stopping the MAOI drug. If you are uncertain if your prescription drug contains an MAOI, consult a health professional before taking this product.

SINUTAB SINUS NO DROWSINESS MAXIMUM STRENGTH
Warner Wellcome Consumer

Dosage Form: caplet, tablet

Active Ingredients: pseudoephedrine hydrochloride (HCl), acetaminophen

Warning: Do not exceed recommended dosage because at higher dosages, nervousness, dizziness, or sleeplessness may occur. Do not take for colds for more than 10 days. If symptoms do not improve or are accompanied by fever that lasts for more than 3 days, or if new symptoms occur, consult a doctor. Do not take this product if you have heart disease, high blood pressure, thyroid disease, diabetes or difficulty in urination due to enlargement of the prostate gland, unless directed by a doctor. If you generally consume 3 or more alcohol-containing drinks per day, you should consult your doctor for advice on when and how you should take this product and other pain relievers. Do not use with other products containing acetaminophen. DRUG INTERACTION PRECAUTION: Do not use this product if you are now taking a prescription monoamine oxidase inhibitor (MAOI) (certain drugs for depression, psychiatric or emotional conditions, or Parkinson's disease) or for 2 weeks after stopping the MAOI drug. If you are uncertain if your prescription drug contains an MAOI, consult a health professional before taking this product.

SLEEP-EZE 3
Whitehall-Robins Healthcare

Dosage Form: tablet

Active Ingredient: diphenhydramine hydrochloride (HCl)

Warning: Do not give to children under 12 years of age. If sleeplessness persists continuously for more than 2 weeks, consult a doctor. Insomnia may be a symptom of serious underlying medical illness. Do not take this product unless directed

by a doctor, if you have breathing problems such as emphysema or chronic bronchitis, or if you have glaucoma, or difficulty in urination due to enlargement of the prostate gland. Avoid alcoholic beverages while taking this product. Do not take this product if you are taking sedatives or tranquilizers without first consulting your doctor.

SLEEPINAL MAXIMUM STRENGTH NIGHT-TIME SLEEP-AID
Thompson Medical Company, Inc.

Dosage Form: capsule, softgel

Active Ingredient: diphenhydramine hydrochloride (HCl)

Warning: Do not give to children under 12 years of age. If sleeplessness persists continuously for more than 2 weeks, consult a doctor. Insomnia may be a symptom of serious underlying medical illness. Do not take this product unless directed by a doctor, if you have breathing problems such as emphysema or chronic bronchitis, or if you have glaucoma, or difficulty in urination due to enlargement of the prostate gland. Avoid alcoholic beverages while taking this product. Do not take this product if you are taking sedatives or tranquilizers without first consulting your doctor.

SOLARCAINE MEDICATED FIRST AID
Schering-Plough HealthCare Products

Dosage Form: aerosol spray

Active Ingredient: benzocaine

Warning: For external use only. Avoid contact with the eyes. If condition worsens, if a rash or irritation develops, if symptoms persist for more than 7 days or clear up and occur again within a few days, discontinue use of this product and consult a doctor. Certain persons can develop allergic reactions to ingredients in this product. Do not use this product if you have a history of allergy to local anesthetics such as procaine, butacaine, benzocaine, or other "caine" anesthetics. Contents under pressure. Do not puncture or incinerate container or place where temperature exceeds 120°F. Flammable mixture; do not use near fire or throw into fire. Use only as directed. Intentional misuse by deliberately concentrating and inhaling the contents can be harmful or fatal.

SOMINEX MAXIMUM STRENGTH
SmithKline Beecham Consumer Health Care, L.P.

Dosage Form: caplet

Active Ingredient: diphenhydramine hydrochloride (HCl)

Warning: Do not give to children under 12 years of age. If sleeplessness persists continuously for more than 2 weeks, consult a doctor. Insomnia may be a symptom of serious underlying medical illness. Do not take this product unless directed by a doctor, if you have breathing problems such as emphysema or chronic bronchitis, or if you have glaucoma, or difficulty in urination due to enlargement of the prostate gland. Avoid alcoholic beverages while taking this product. Do not take this product if you are taking sedatives or tranquilizers without first consulting your doctor.

SPEC-T SORE THROAT COUGH SUPPRESSANT LOZENGES
Apothecon, Division of Bristol-Myers Squibb Company

Dosage Form: lozenge

Active Ingredient: benzocaine

Warning: A severe or persistent sore throat that is accompanied by a high fever, headache, rash, swelling, nausea or vomiting may be serious. Consult your doctor promptly. A persistent cough may be a sign of a serious condition. Persons with a high fever or persistent cough should not use this preparation without consulting a doctor. Do not use for more than 2 days unless directed by a doctor. Certain persons can develop allergic reactions to ingredients in this product. Do not use this product if you have a history of allergy to local anesthetics such as procaine, butacaine, benzocaine, or other "caine" anesthetics. DRUG INTERACTION PRECAUTION: Do not use this product if you are now taking a prescription monoamine oxidase inhibitor (MAOI) (certain drugs for depression, psychiatric or emotional conditions, or Parkinson's disease) or for 2 weeks after stopping the MAOI drug. If you are uncertain if your prescription drug contains an MAOI, consult a health professional before taking this product.

STING-EZE
Wisconsin Pharmacal Company, Inc.

Dosage Form: drops

Active Ingredients: camphor, phenol, benzocaine, diphenhydramine hydrochloride (HCl)

Warning: For external use only. Avoid contact with the eyes. If accidental eye contact is made, flush freely with water for 15 minutes and call a doctor.

STING-KILL
Kiwi Brands Inc.

Dosage Form: liquid

Active Ingredients: benzocaine, menthol

Warning: For external use only. Avoid contact with the eyes. If condition worsens, or if symptoms persist for more than 7 days, discontinue use of this product and consult a doctor. Do not use on children under 2 years of age except under the advice and supervision of a doctor.

STRI-DEX ANTIBACTERIAL CLEANSING BAR
Blistex Inc.

Dosage Form: cleansing bar

Active Ingredient: triclosan

Warning: Do not use this product on infants under 6 months of age. For external use only. Avoid contact with eyes. If contact occurs, flush thoroughly with water. Using other topical acne medications at the same time or immediately following use of this product may increase dryness or irritation of the skin. If this occurs, only one medication should be used unless directed by a doctor.

STRI-DEX CLEAR GEL
Blistex Inc.

Dosage Form: gel

Active Ingredient: salicylic acid

Warning: For external use only. Keep away from eyes, lips and other mucous membranes. If contact with eyes occurs, flush thoroughly with water. Using other topical acne medications at the same time or immediately following use of this product may increase dryness or irritaion of the skin. If this occurs, only one medication should be used unless directed by a doctor. Persons who are sensitive to or have a known allergy to salicylic acid should not use this medication. If irritation, or excessive dryness, and/or peeling occurs, reduce frequency of use or dosage. If excessive itching, dryness, redness or swelling occurs discontinue use. If these symptoms persist consult a doctor promptly.

STRI-DEX PADS MAXIMUM STRENGTH
Blistex Inc.

Dosage Form: pad

Active Ingredient: salicylic acid

Warning: For external use only. Keep away from eyes, lips, and other mucous membranes.Using other topical acne medications at the same time or immediately following use of this product may increase dryness or irritaion of the skin. If this occurs, only one medication should be used unless directed by a doctor. Persons who are sensitive to or have a known allergy to salicylic acid should not use this medication. If irritation, or excessive dryness, and/or peeling occurs, reduce frequency of use or dosage. If excessive itching, dryness, redness or swelling occurs, discontinue use. If these symptoms persist, consult a doctor promptly.

SUCRETS 4-HOUR COUGH SUPPRESSANT
SmithKline Beecham Consumer Health Care, L.P.

Dosage Form: lozenge

Active Ingredients: dextromethorphan hydrobromide, menthol

Warning: A persistent cough may be a sign of a serious condition. If cough persists for more than 1 week, tends to recur, or is accompanied by a fever, rash or persistent headache, consult a doctor. Do not take this product for persistent or chronic cough such as occurs with smoking, asthma, emphysema, or if cough is accompanied by excessive phlegm (mucous) unless directed by a doctor. DRUG INTERACTION PRE-CAUTION: Do not use this product if you are now taking a prescription monoamine oxidase inhibitor (MAOI) (certain drugs for depression, psychiatric or emotional conditions, or Parkinson's disease) or for 2 weeks after stopping the MAOI drug. If you are uncertain if your prescription drug contains an MAOI, consult a health professional before taking this product.

SUCRETS CHILDREN'S SORE THROAT LOZENGES
SmithKline Beecham Consumer Health Care, L.P.

Dosage Form: lozenge

Active Ingredient: dyclonine hydrochloride (HCl)

Warning: If sore throat is severe, persists for more than 2 days, is accompanied or followed by fever, headache, rash, swelling, nausea or vomiting, consult a doctor promptly. If sore mouth symptoms do not improve in 7 days, or if irritation, pain, or redness persists or worsens, see your dentist or doctor promptly. Do not exceed recommended dosage.

SUCRETS MAXIMUM STRENGTH
SmithKline Beecham Consumer Health Care, L.P.

Dosage Form: lozenge

Active Ingredient: dyclonine hydrochloride (HCl)

Warning: Do not exceed recommended dosage. If sore throat is severe, persists for more than 2 days, is accompanied or followed by a fever, headache, rash, swelling, nausea or vomiting, consult a doctor promptly. If sore mouth symptoms do not improve in 7 days, or if irritation, pain, or redness persists or worsens, see your dentist or doctor promptly. Do not exceed recommended dosage.

SUDAFED CHILDREN'S NASAL DECONGESTANT
Warner Wellcome Consumer

Dosage Form: liquid

Active Ingredient: pseudoephedrine hydrochloride (HCl)

Warning: Do not exceed recommended dosage because at higher dosages, nervousness, dizziness, or sleeplessness may occur. If symptoms do not improve within 7 days or are accompanied by a fever, consult a doctor. Do not take this product if you have heart disease, high blood pressure, diabetes, thyroid disease, or difficulty in urination due to enlargement of the prostate gland unless directed by a doctor. DRUG INTERACTION PRE-CAUTION: Do not use this product if you are now taking a prescription monoamine oxidase inhibitor (MAOI) (certain drugs for depression, psychiatric or emotional conditions, or Parkinson's disease) or for 2 weeks after stopping the MAOI drug. If you are uncertain if your prescription drug contains an MAOI, consult a health professional before taking this product.

SUDAFED COLD & ALLERGY
Warner Wellcome Consumer

Dosage Form: tablet

Active Ingredients: pseudoephedrine hydrochloride (HCl), chlorpheniramine maleate

Warning: Do not exceed recommended dosage because at higher dosages, nervousness, dizziness, or sleeplessness may occur. If symptoms do not improve within 7 days or are accompanied by a fever, consult a doctor. Do not take this product if you have a breathing problem such as emphysema or chronic bronchitis, or if you have heart disease, high blood pressure, diabetes, thyroid disease, glaucoma or difficulty in urination due to enlargement of the prostate gland unless directed by a doctor. May cause excitability especially in children. May cause drowsiness; alcohol, sedatives, and tranquilizers may increase its drowsiness effect. Avoid alcoholic beverages while taking this product. Do not take this product if you are taking sedatives or tranquilizers without first consulting your doctor. Use caution while driving a motor vehicle or operating machinery. DRUG INTERACTION PRECAUTION: Do not use this product if you are now taking a prescription monoamine oxidase inhibitor (MAOI) (certain drugs

for depression, psychiatric or emotional conditions, or Parkinson's disease) or for 2 weeks after stopping the MAOI drug. If you are uncertain if your prescription drug contains an MAOI, consult a health professional before taking this product.

SUDAFED NASAL DECONGESTANT
Warner Wellcome Consumer

Dosage Form: tablet

Active Ingredient: pseudoephedrine hydrochloride (HCl)

Warning: Do not exceed recommended dosage because at higher dosages nervousness, dizziness or sleeplessness may occur. If symptoms do not improve within 7 days or are accompanied by a fever, consult a doctor. Do not take this product if you have heart disease, high blood pressure, diabetes, thyroid disease, or difficulty in urination due to enlargement of the prostate gland unless directed by a doctor. DRUG INTERACTION PRECAUTION: Do not use this product if you are now taking a prescription monoamine oxidase inhibitor (MAOI) (certain drugs for depression, psychiatric or emotional conditions, or Parkinson's disease) or for 2 weeks after stopping the MAOI drug. If you are uncertain if your prescription drug contains an MAOI, consult a health professional before taking this product.

SURFAK STOOL SOFTENER
Pharmacia & Upjohn, Inc.

Dosage Form: liqui-gels

Active Ingredient: docusate calcium

Warning: Do not use this product when abdominal pain, nausea or vomiting are present, unless directed by a doctor. Laxative products should not be used for a period longer than 1 week unless directed by a doctor. If you have noticed a sudden change in bowel habits that persists over a period of 2 weeks, consult a doctor before using a laxative. Rectal bleeding or failure to have a bowel movement after use of a laxative may indicate a serious condition. Discontinue use and consult a doctor. DRUG INTERACTION PRECAUTION: Do not take this product if you are presently taking mineral oil, unless directed by a doctor.

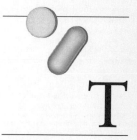

TAGAMET HB 200
SmithKline Beecham Consumer Health Care, L.P.

Dosage Form: tablet

Active Ingredient: cimetidine

Warning: Consult your doctor if you are taking theophylline (oral asthma medicine), warfarin (blood thinning medicine), or phenytoin (seizure medicine) before taking TAGAMET HB

200. If you are not sure whether your medication contains one of these drugs or have any other questions about medicines you are taking, call our consumer affairs specialist at 1–800–482–4394. Do not take the maximum daily dosage for more than 2 weeks continuously except under the advice and supervision of a doctor. If you have trouble swallowing, or persistent abdominal pain, see your doctor promptly. You may have a serious condition that may need different treatment.

TANAC NO STING
Del Pharmaceuticals, Inc.

Dosage Form: liquid

Active Ingredient: benzocaine

Warning: If the condition for which this preparation is used persists or if a rash or irritation develops, discontinue use and consult a doctor. Use as indicated but not for more than 5 consecutive days. Not for prolonged use. Avoid getting into eyes. Certain persons can develop allergic reactions to ingredients in this product. Do not use this product if you have a history of allergy to local anesthetics such as procaine, butacaine, benzocaine, or other "caine" anesthetics.

TAVIST-1
Sandoz North American Consumer Pharmaceuticals*

Dosage Form: tablet

Active Ingredient: clemastine fumarate

Warning: May cause excitability especially in children. Do not take this product if you have asthma, glaucoma, emphysema, chronic pulmonary disease, shortness of breath, difficulty in breathing, or difficulty in urination due to enlargement of the prostate gland unless directed by a doctor. May cause drowsiness; alcohol, sedatives, and tranquilizers may increase its drowsiness effect. Avoid alcoholic beverages while taking this product. Do not take this product if you are taking sedatives or tranquilizers without first consulting your doctor. Use caution while driving a motor vehicle or operating machinery.

TAVIST-D
Sandoz North American Consumer Pharmaceuticals*

Dosage Form: tablet

Active Ingredient: phenylpropanolamine hydrochloride (HCl), clemastine fumarate

Warning: Do not exceed recommended dosage because at higher dosages, nervousness, dizziness, or sleeplessness may occur. Do not take this product for more than 7 days. If symptoms do not improve or are accompanied by fever, consult a doctor. Do not take this product if you have asthma, diabetes, glaucoma, heart disease, high blood pressure, thyroid disease, emphysema, chronic pulmonary disease, shortness of breath, difficulty in breathing, or difficulty in urination due to enlargement of the prostate gland unless directed by a doctor. May cause excitability especially in children. May cause drowsiness; alcohol, sedatives, and tranquilizers may increase the drowsiness effect. Avoid alcoholic beverages while taking this product. Do not take this product if you are

taking sedatives or tranquilizers without first consulting your doctor. Use caution when driving a motor vehicle or operating machinery. Do not take this product if you are taking another medication containing phenylpropanolamine. DRUG INTERACTION PRECAUTION: Do not use this product if you are now taking a prescription drug for high blood pressure without first consulting your doctor or if you are now taking a prescription monoamine oxidase inhibitor (MAOI) (certain drugs for depression, psychiatric or emotional conditions, or Parkinson's disease) or for 2 weeks after stopping the MAOI drug. If you are uncertain if your prescription drug contains an MAOI, consult a health professional before taking this product.

TEARS NATURALE
Alcon Laboratories, Inc.

Dosage Form: drops

Active Ingredients: hydroxypropyl methylcellulose, dextran 70

Warning: To avoid contamination, do not touch tip of container to any surface. Replace cap after using. If you experience eye pain, changes in vision, continued redness or irritation of the eye or if the condition worsens or persists for more than 72 hours, discontinue use and consult a doctor. If solution changes color or becomes cloudy, do not use. Remove contact lenses before using.

TEGRIN DANDRUFF SHAMPOO
Block Drug

Dosage Form: shampoo

Active Ingredient: coal tar solution

Warning: For external use only. Avoid contact with the eyes. If contact occurs, rinse eyes thoroughly with water. If condition worsens or does not improve after regular use of this product as directed, consult a doctor. Use caution in exposing skin to sunlight after applying this product. It may increase tendency to sunburn for up to 24 hours after application. Do not use for prolonged periods without consulting a doctor. Do not use this product with other forms of psoriasis therapy, such as ultraviolet radiation or prescription drugs, unless directed by a doctor.

TEGRIN-LT LICE TREATMENT SHAMPOO/CONDITIONER
Block Drug

Dosage Form: shampoo, conditioner

Active Ingredients: piperonyl butoxide, pyrethrum extract

Warning: Use with caution on persons allergic to ragweed. For external use only. Do not use near the eyes or permit contact with mucous membranes such as inside the nose, mouth, or vagina, as irritation may occur. Keep out of eyes when rinsing hair. *Adults and children:* Close eyes tightly and do not open eyes until product is rinsed out. Also, protect children's eyes with washcloth, towel or other suitable material, or by similar method. If product gets into the eyes, immediately flush with water. If skin irritation or infection is present or develops, discontinue use and consult a doctor. Consult a doctor if infestation of eyebrows or eyelashes occurs.

TEMPRA 2
Bristol-Myers Products

Dosage Form: syrup

Active Ingredient: acetaminophen

Warning: Contact your doctor if fever continues for more than 3 days (72 hours) or pain continues for more than 5 days. Do not use with other products containing acetaminophen. Do not use if carton is open or tamper resistent neck band on bottle is broken or missing.

THERAFLU FLU AND COLD MEDICINE ORIGINAL FORMULA
Sandoz North American Consumer Pharmaceuticals*

Dosage Form: individual packet (powder)

Active Ingredients: pseudoephedrine hydrochloride (HCl), chlorpheniramine maleate, acetaminophen

Warning: Do not take this product for more than 7 days. If symptoms do not improve or are accompanied by a fever that lasts for more than 3 days or recurs, or if new symptoms occur, consult a doctor before continuing use. If pain or fever persists, or gets worse, or if redness or swelling is present, consult a doctor. If sore throat is severe, persists for more than 2 days, or is accompanied or followed by a fever, headache, rash, nausea or vomiting, consult a doctor promptly. Do not take this product if you have a breathing problem such as emphysema or chronic bronchitis, or if you have heart disease, high blood pressure, diabetes, thyroid disease, glaucoma, or difficulty in urination due to enlargement of the prostate gland unless directed by a doctor. May cause excitability especially in children. May cause drowsiness; alcohol, sedatives, and tranquilizers may increase its drowsiness effect. Avoid alcoholic beverages while taking this product. Do not take this product if you are taking sedatives or tranquilizers without first consulting your doctor. Use caution while driving a motor vehicle or operating machinery. Do not use with other products containing acetaminophen. DRUG INTERACTION PRECAUTION: Do not use this product if you are now taking a prescription monoamine oxidase inhibitor (MAOI) (certain drugs for depression, psychiatric or emotional conditions, or Parkinson's disease) or for 2 weeks after stopping the MAOI drug. If you are uncertain if your prescription drug contains an MAOI, consult a health professional before taking this product.

THERAFLU FLU COLD & COUGH MEDICINE NIGHTTIME
Sandoz North American Consumer Pharmaceuticals*

Dosage Form: individual packet (powder), caplet

Active Ingredients: pseudoephedrine hydrochloride (HCl), chlorpheniramine maleate, acetaminophen, dextromethorphan hydrobromide

Warning: Do not exceed recommended dosage. If nervousness, dizziness, or sleeplessness occur, discontinue use and consult a doctor. If symptoms do not improve within 7 days or are accompanied by a fever that lasts for more than 3 days, or if new symptoms occur, or if redness or swelling is present, consult a doctor. These could be signs of a serious condition. If sore throat is severe, persists for more than 2 days, or is accompanied or followed by a fever, headache, rash, nausea or vomiting, consult a doctor promptly. If cough persists for more than 1 week, tends to recur, or is accompanied by a fever, rash or persistent headache, consult a doctor. A persistent cough may be a sign of a serious condition. Do not take this product for persistent or chronic cough such as occurs with smoking, asthma, or emphysema, or if cough is accompanied by excessive phlegm (mucous) unless directed by a doctor. Do not take this product, if you have a breathing problem such as emphysema or chronic bronchitis, or if you have glaucoma, high blood pressure, heart disease, thyroid disease, diabetes or difficulty in urination due to the enlargement of the prostate gland, without first consulting a doctor. May cause excitability especially in children. May cause marked drowsiness; alcohol, sedatives, and tranquilizers may increase its drowsiness effect. Avoid alcoholic beverages while taking this product. Do not take this product if you are taking sedatives or tranquilizers without first consulting your doctor. Use caution while driving a motor vehicle or operating machinery. Do not use with other products containing acetaminophen. DRUG INTERACTION PRECAUTION: Do not use this product if you are now taking a prescription monoamine oxidase inhibitor (MAOI) (certain drugs for depression, psychiatric or emotional conditions, or Parkinson's disease) or for 2 weeks after stopping the MAOI drug. If you are uncertain if your prescription drug contains an MAOI, consult a health professional before taking this product.

THERA-GESIC EXTRA STRENGTH
Mission Pharmaceutical Company

Dosage Form: cream

Active Ingredients: methyl salicylate, menthol

Warning: For external use only. Use only as directed. Avoid contact with eyes, mucous membranes. If skin redness or irritation develops, or pain lasts for more than 10 days, or clears up and occurs again within a few days, discontinue use and consult a doctor. If prone to allergic reaction to aspirin or salicylates, consult a doctor before using. Do not apply to wounds, or to damaged, broken (open) or irritated skin. Do not bandage tightly. Do not use with a heating pad. Do not swallow. If swallowed, induce vomiting and call a doctor. Contact a doctor before giving this medicine to children, including teenagers, with chicken pox or flu.

THERAPEUTIC MINERAL ICE
Bristol-Myers Products

Dosage Form: gel

Active Ingredient: menthol

Warning: For external use only. Use only as directed. Avoid contact with eyes and mucous membranes. Do not use with other ointments, creams, sprays, or liniments. If skin redness or irritation develops, if condition worsens, or does not improve within 7 days, or clears up and occurs again

within a few days, discontinue use and consult a doctor. Do not apply to wounds, or to damaged, broken (open) or irritated skin. Do not bandage tightly. Do not use with heating pads or heating devices. If you have sensitive skin, consult a doctor before use.

TINACTIN ANTIFUNGAL
Schering-Plough HealthCare Products

Dosage Form: solution, cream, powder, aerosol spray

Active Ingredient: tolnaftate

Warning: For external use only. Do not use on children under 2 years of age unless directed by a doctor. Avoid contact with the eyes. If irritation occurs or if there is no improvement within 4 weeks (for athlete's foot or ringworm) or within 2 weeks (for jock itch), discontinue use and consult a doctor or pharmacist. *For liquid aerosol, powder aerosol and powder spray only:* Avoid inhaling. Avoid contact with the eyes and other mucous membranes. Contents under pressure. Do not puncture or incinerate. Flammable mixture, do not use while smoking or near fire or flame. Do not expose to heat or temperatures above 49°C (120°F). Use only as directed. Intentional misuse by deliberately concentrating and inhaling the contents can be harmful or fatal.

TING ANTIFUNGAL
Ciba Self-Medication, Inc. *

Dosage Form: aerosol spray powder, cream, powder, aerosol spray

Active Ingredient: tolnaftate

Warning: For external use only. Do not use on children under 2 years of age unless directed by a doctor. Avoid contact with the eyes. If irritation occurs or if there is no improvement within 4 weeks for athlete's foot or within 2 weeks for jock itch, discontinue use and consult a doctor. Use only as directed. *For sprays only:* Avoid inhaling. Avoid contact with the eye or other mucous membranes. Contents under pressure; do not puncture or incinerate. Flammable mixture, do not use near fire or flame. Do not expose to heat or temperatures above 49°C (120°F). Use only as directed. Intentional misuse by deliberately concentrating and inhaling contents can be harmful or fatal.

TISIT
Pfeiffer Pharmaceuticals, Inc.

Dosage Form: shampoo

Active Ingredients: piperonyl butoxide, pyrethrins

Warning: Use with caution on persons allergic to ragweed. For external use only. Do not use near the eyes or permit contact with mucous membranes such as inside the nose, mouth, or vagina, as irritation may occur. Keep out of eyes when rinsing hair. *Adults and children:* Close eyes tightly and do not open eyes until product is rinsed out. Also, protect children's eyes with washcloth, towel or other suitable material, or by similar method. If product gets into the eyes, immediately flush with water. If skin irritation or infection is present or develops, discontinue use and consult a doctor. Consult a doctor if infestation of eyebrows or eyelashes occurs.

TOLU-SED DM
Scherer Laboratories, Inc.

Dosage Form: liquid

Active Ingredients: guaifenesin, dextromethorphan hydrobromide

Warning: A persistent cough may be a sign of a serious condition. If cough persists for more than 1 week, tends to recur, or is accompanied by a fever, rash or persistent headache, consult a doctor. Do not take this product for persistent or chronic cough such as occurs with smoking, asthma, chronic bronchitis, or emphysema, or where cough is accompanied by excessive phlegm (mucous) unless directed by a doctor. DRUG INTERACTION PRECAUTION: Do not use this product if you are now taking a prescription monoamine oxidase inhibitor (MAOI) (certain drugs for depression, psychiatric or emotional conditions, or Parkinson's disease) or for 2 weeks after stopping the MAOI drug. If you are uncertain if your prescription drug contains an MAOI, consult a health professional before taking this product.

**TRIAMINIC AM
NON-DROWSY DECONGESTANT**
*Sandoz North American
Consumer Pharmaceuticals* *

Dosage Form: syrup

Active Ingredients: pseudoephedrine hydrochloride (HCl), dextromethorphan hydrobromide

Warning: Do not exceed recommended dosage because at higher dosages, nervousness, dizziness, or sleeplessness may occur. If symptoms do not improve within 7 days or are accompanied by a fever, consult a doctor. Do not take this product if you have heart disease, high blood pressure, diabetes, thyroid disease, or difficulty in urination due to enlargement of the prostate gland unless directed by a doctor. DRUG INTERACTION PRECAUTION: Do not use this product if you are now taking a prescription monoamine oxidase inhibitor (MAOI) (certain drugs for depression, psychiatric or emotional conditions, or Parkinson's disease) or for 2 weeks after stopping the MAOI drug. If you are uncertain if your prescription drug contains an MAOI, consult a health professional before taking this product.

**TRIAMINIC NIGHT TIME
MAXIMUM STRENGTH**
*Sandoz North American
Consumer Pharmaceuticals* *

Dosage Form: liquid

Active Ingredients: pseudoephedrine hydrochloride (HCl), chlorpheniramine maleate, dextromethorphan hydrobromide

Warning: Do not exceed recommended dosage because at higher dosages, nervousness, dizziness, or sleeplessness may occur. If symptoms do not improve within 7 days or are accompanied by a fever, consult a doctor. A persistent cough may be a sign of a serious condition. If cough persists for more than 1 week, tends to recur, or is accompanied by a fever, rash or persistent headache, consult a doctor. Do not take this product for persistent or chronic cough such as occurs with smoking, asthma, chronic bronchitis, or emphysema, or if cough is accompanied by excessive phlegm (mucous) unless directed by a doctor. Do not take this product if you have a breathing problem such as emphysema or chronic bronchitis, or if you have heart disease, high blood pressure, diabetes, thyroid disease, glaucoma, or difficulty in urination due to enlargement of the prostate gland unless directed by a doctor. May cause excitability especially in children. May cause drowsiness; alcohol, sedatives, and tranquilizers may increase its drowsiness effect. Avoid alcoholic beverages while taking this product. Do not take this product if you are taking sedatives or tranquilizers without first consulting your doctor. Use caution while driving a motor vehicle or operating machinery. DRUG INTERACTION PRECAUTION: Do not use this product if you are now taking a prescription monoamine oxidase inhibitor (MAOI) (certain drugs for depression, psychiatric or emotional conditions, or Parkinson's disease) or for 2 weeks after stopping the MAOI drug. If you are uncertain if your prescription drug contains an MAOI, consult a health professional before taking this product.

TRIAMINIC SORE THROAT, THROAT PAIN & COUGH
*Sandoz North American Consumer Pharmaceuticals**

Dosage Form: liquid

Active Ingredients: pseudoephedrine hydrochloride (HCl), acetaminophen, dextromethorphan hydrobromide

Warning: Do not exceed recommended dosage. If nervousness, dizziness, or sleeplessness occur, discontinue use and consult a doctor. Do not take this product for more than 7 days (for adults) or 5 days (for children). Do not take for sore throat pain for more than 2 days, and for fever for more than 3 days. If pain or fever persists, gets worse, if new symptoms occur, or if redness or swelling is present, consult a doctor. These could be signs of a serious condition. If sore throat is severe, persists for more than 2 days, or is accompanied or followed by a fever, headache, rash, nausea or vomiting, consult a doctor promptly. If symptoms do not improve within 7 days or are accompanied by a fever, consult a doctor. A persistent cough may be a sign of a serious condition. If cough persists for more than 1 week, tends to recur, or is accompanied by a rash, persistent headache, fever that lasts for more than 3 days, or if new symptoms occur, consult a doctor. Do not take this product for persistent or chronic cough such as occurs with smoking, asthma, chronic bronchitis, or emphysema, or where cough is accompanied by excessive phlegm (mucous) unless directed by a doctor. Do not take this product if you have heart disease, high blood pressure, diabetes, thyroid disease, or difficulty in urination due to enlargement of the prostate gland unless directed by a doctor. DRUG INTERACTION PRECAUTION: Do not use this product if you are now taking a prescription monoamine oxidase inhibitor (MAOI) (certain drugs for depression, psychiatric or emotional conditions, or Parkinson's disease) or for 2 weeks after stopping the MAOI drug. If you are uncertain if your prescription drug contains an MAOI,

consult a health professional before taking this product.

TRIAMINIC SYRUP COLD & ALLERGY
*Sandoz North American Consumer Pharmaceuticals**

Dosage Form: syrup

Active Ingredients: phenylpropanolamine hydrochloride (HCl), chlorpheniramine maleate

Warning: Do not exceed recommended dosage because at higher dosages, nervousness, dizziness, or sleeplessness may occur. If symptoms do not improve within 7 days or are accompanied by a fever, consult a doctor. Do not take this product if you have a breathing problem such as emphysema or chronic bronchitis, heart disease, high blood pressure, diabetes, thyroid disease, or if you have glaucoma or difficulty in urination due to enlargement of the prostate gland unless directed by a doctor. May cause excitability especially in children. May cause drowsiness; alcohol, sedatives, and tranquilizers may increase its drowsiness effect. Avoid alcoholic beverages while taking this product. Do not take this product if you are taking sedatives or tranquilizers without first consulting your doctor. Use caution while driving a motor vehicle or operating machinery. Do not use if you are presently taking another medication containing phenylpropanolamine, unless directed by a doctor. DRUG INTERACTION PRECAUTION: Do not use this product if you are now taking a prescription monoamine oxidase inhibitor (MAOI) (certain drugs for depression, psychiatric or emotional conditions, or Parkinson's disease) or for 2 weeks after stopping the MAOI drug. If you are uncertain if your prescription drug contains an MAOI, consult a health professional before taking this product.

TRIAMINIC TRIAMINICOL COLD & COUGH
*Sandoz North American Consumer Pharmaceuticals**

Dosage Form: liquid

Active Ingredients: phenylpropanolamine hydrochloride (HCl), chlorpheniramine maleate, dextromethorphan hydrobromide

Warning: Do not exceed recommended dosage because at higher dosages, nervousness, dizziness, or sleeplessness may occur. If symptoms do not improve within 7 days or are accompanied by a fever, consult a doctor. If cough persists for more than 1 week, tends to recur, or is accompanied by a fever, rash or persistent headache, consult a doctor. Do not take this product for persistent or chronic cough such as occurs with smoking, asthma, chronic bronchitis, or emphysema, or if cough is accompanied by excessive phlegm (mucous) unless directed by a doctor. Do not take this product if you have a breathing problem such as emphysema or chronic bronchitis, or if you have heart disease, high blood pressure, diabetes, thyroid disease, glaucoma, or difficulty in urination due to enlargement of the prostate gland unless directed by a doctor. May cause marked drowsiness; alcohol, sedatives, and tranquilizers may increase its drowsiness effect. Avoid alcoholic beverages while taking this product. Do

not take this product while taking sedatives or tranquilizers without first consulting your doctor. Use caution while driving a motor vehicle or operating machinery. Do not take this product if you are presently taking another product containing phenylpropanolamine. DRUG INTERACTION PRECAUTION: Do not use this product if you are now taking a prescription monoamine oxidase inhibitor (MAOI) (certain drugs for depression, psychiatric or emotional conditions, or Parkinson's disease) or for 2 weeks after stopping the MAOI drug. If you are uncertain if your prescription drug contains an MAOI, consult a health professional before taking this product.

TRIAMINICIN COLD, ALLERGY, SINUS MEDICINE
*Sandoz North American Consumer Pharmaceuticals**

Dosage Form: tablet

Active Ingredients: phenylpropanolamine hydrochloride (HCl), chlorpheniramine maleate, acetaminophen

Warning: Do not exceed recommended dosage because at higher dosages, nervousness, dizziness, or sleeplessness may occur. Do not take for pain for more than 7 days or for fever for more than 3 days unless directed by a doctor. If pain or fever persists, or gets worse, if new symptoms occur, or if redness or swelling is present, consult a doctor because these could be signs of a serious condition. Do not take this product if you have a breathing problem such as emphysema or chronic bronchitis, or if you have heart disease, high blood pressure, diabetes, thyroid disease, glaucoma or difficulty in urination due to enlargement of the prostate gland unless directed by a doctor. May cause excitability especially in children. May cause drowsiness. Alcohol, sedatives, and tranquilizers may increase its drowsiness effect. Avoid alcoholic beverages while taking this product. Do not take this product while taking sedatives or tranquilizers without first consulting your doctor. Use caution while driving a motor vehicle or operating machinery. Do not take this product if you are taking an appetite-controlling medication containing phenylpropanolamine without first consulting your doctor. Do not use with other products containing acetaminophen. DRUG INTERACTION PRECAUTION: Do not use this product if you are now taking a prescription monoamine oxidase inhibitor (MAOI) (certain drugs for depression, psychiatric or emotional conditions, or Parkinson's disease) or for 2 weeks after stopping the MAOI drug. If you are uncertain if your prescription drug contains an MAOI, consult a health professional before taking this product.

TRIPTONE
Del Pharmaceuticals, Inc.

Dosage Form: tablet

Active Ingredient: dimenhydrinate

Warning: Do not give to children under 2 years of age unless directed by a doctor. Do not take this product, if you have breathing problems such as emphysema, or chronic bronchitis, or if you have glaucoma, or difficulty in urination due to enlargement of the prostate gland, unless directed by a doctor. May cause drowsiness; alcohol, sedatives, and tranquilizers may increase its drowsiness effect. Avoid alcoholic beverages while taking this product. Do not take this product if you are taking sedatives or tranquilizers without first consulting your doctor. Use caution when driving a motor vehicle or operating machinery. Not for frequent or prolonged use, except on advice of a doctor. Do not exceed recommended dosage.

TRONOLANE
Ross Products/Abbott Laboratories

Dosage Form: cream

Active Ingredient: pramoxine hydrochloride (HCl)

Warning: If condition worsens or does not improve within 7 days, consult a doctor. If the symptom being treated does not subside, or if redness, irritation, swelling, pain or other symptoms develop or increase, discontinue use and consult a doctor. Do not exceed the recommended daily dosage, unless directed by a doctor. In case of bleeding, consult a doctor promptly. Do not put this product into the rectum by using fingers or any mechanical device or applicator. Certain persons can develop allergic reactions to the ingredients in this product.

TUCKS MEDICATED PADS
Warner Wellcome Consumer

Dosage Form: pad

Active Ingredient: witch hazel

Warning: If condition worsens or does not improve within 7 days, consult a doctor. Do not exceed the recommended daily dosage, unless directed by a doctor. In case of bleeding, consult a doctor promptly. Do not put this product into the rectum by using fingers or any mechanical device or applicator.

TUMS E-X EXTRA STRENGTH
SmithKline Beecham
Consumer Health Care, L.P.

Dosage Form: chewable tablet

Active Ingredient: calcium carbonate

Warning: Do not take more than 10 tablets in a 24 hour period or use the maximum strength of this product for more than 2 weeks, except under the advice and supervision of a doctor. If symptoms persist for more than 2 weeks stop using this product and see a doctor. DRUG INTERACTION PRECAUTION: Antacids may interact with certain prescription drugs. If you are presently taking a prescription drug, do not take this product without checking with your doctor or health professional.

TYLENOL ALLERGY SINUS MAXIMUM STRENGTH
McNeil Consumer Products Company

Dosage Form: gelcap, caplet, geltab

Active Ingredients: pseudoephedrine hydrochloride (HCl), chlorpheniramine maleate, acetaminophen

Warning: Do not exceed recommended dosage because at higher dosages, nervousness, dizziness, or sleeplessness may occur. Do not take for pain for more than 7 days or for fever for more

than 3 days unless directed by a doctor. If pain or fever persists, or gets worse, if new symptoms occur, or if redness or swelling is present, consult a doctor because these could be signs of a serious condition. Do not take this product if you have a breathing problem such as emphysema or chronic bronchitis, heart disease, high blood pressure, diabetes, thyroid disease, or if you have glaucoma or difficulty in urination due to enlargement of the prostate gland unless directed by a doctor. May cause excitability especially in children. May cause drowsiness; alcohol, sedatives, and tranquilizers may increase its drowsiness effect. Avoid alcoholic beverages while taking this product. Do not take this product if you are taking sedatives or tranquilizers without first consulting your doctor. Use caution while driving a motor vehicle or operating machinery. If you generally consume 3 or more alcohol-containing drinks per day, you should consult your physician for advice on when and how you should take this product and other pain relievers. Do not use with other products containing acetaminophen. DRUG INTERACTION PRECAUTION: Do not use this product if you are now taking a prescription monoamine oxidase inhibitor (MAOI) (certain drugs for depression, psychiatric or emotional conditions, or Parkinson's disease) or for 2 weeks after stopping the MAOI drug. If you are uncertain if your prescription drug contains an MAOI, consult a health professional before taking this product.

TYLENOL ALLERGY SINUS NIGHTTIME MAXIMUM STRENGTH
McNeil Consumer Products Company

Dosage Form: caplet

Active Ingredients: pseudoephedrine hydrochloride (HCl), diphenhydramine hydrochloride (HCl), acetaminophen

Warning: Do not exceed recommended dosage because at higher dosages, nervousness, dizziness, or sleeplessness may occur. Do not take for pain for more than 7 days or for fever for more than 3 days unless directed by a doctor. If pain or fever persists, or gets worse, if new symptoms occur, or if redness or swelling is present, consult a doctor because these could be signs of a serious condition. Do not take this product if you have a breathing problem such as emphysema or chronic bronchitis, heart disease, high blood pressure, diabetes, thyroid disease, or if you have glaucoma or difficulty in urination due to enlargement of the prostate gland unless directed by a doctor. May cause excitability especially in children. May cause drowsiness; alcohol, sedatives, and tranquilizers may increase its drowsiness effect. Avoid alcoholic beverages while taking this product. Do not take this product if you are taking sedatives or tranquilizers without first consulting your doctor. Use caution while driving a motor vehicle or operating machinery. If you generally consume 3 or more alcohol-containing drinks per day, you should consult your physician for advice on when and how you should take this product and other pain relievers. Do not use with other products containing acetaminophen. DRUG INTERACTION PRECAUTION: Do not use this product if you

are now taking a prescription monoamine oxidase inhibitor (MAOI) (certain drugs for depression, psychiatric or emotional conditions, or Parkinson's disease) or for 2 weeks after stopping the MAOI drug. If you are uncertain if your prescription drug contains an MAOI, consult a health professional before taking this product.

TYLENOL CHILDREN'S
McNeil Consumer Products Company

Dosage Form: suspension liquid, elixir, chewable tablets, caplet

Active Ingredient: acetaminophen

Warning: Contact your doctor if fever persists for more than 3 days (72 hours) or if pain continues for more than 5 days. Not a USP elixir. Do not use with other products containing acetaminophen. Do not use if imprinted carton overwrap is broken or missing or if carton is open. Do not use if printed plastic bottle wrap or printed foil inner seal is broken.

TYLENOL CHILDREN'S COLD MULTI SYMPTOM
McNeil Consumer Products Company

Dosage Form: chewable tablet, liquid

Active Ingredients: pseudoephedrine hydrochloride (HCl), chlorpheniramine maleate, acetaminophen

Warning: Do not exceed recommended dosage because at higher dosages, nervousness, dizziness, or sleeplessness may occur. Do not take for pain for more than 5 days or for fever for more than 3 days unless directed by a doctor. If pain or fever persists, or gets worse, if new symptoms occur, or if redness or swelling is present, consult a doctor because these could be signs of a serious condition. If sore throat is severe, persists for more than 2 days, is accompanied by or followed by fever, headache, nausea or vomiting, consult a doctor promptly. Do not give this product to a child who has a breathing problem such as chronic bronchitis, or who has heart disease, high blood pressure, diabetes, thyroid disease, or glaucoma unless directed by a doctor. May cause excitability especially in children. May cause drowsiness; sedatives, and tranquilizers may increase its drowsiness effect. Do not give this product to a child who is taking sedatives or tranquilizers without first consulting your doctor. Do not use with other products containing acetaminophen. DRUG INTERACTION PRECAUTION: Do not give this product to a child who is taking a prescription monoamine oxidase inhibitor (MAOI) (certain drugs for depression, psychiatric or emotional conditions) or for 2 weeks after stopping the MAOI drug. If you are uncertain if your child's prescription drug contains an MAOI, consult a health professional before taking this product.

TYLENOL CHILDREN'S COLD MULTI SYMPTOM PLUS COUGH
McNeil Consumer Products Company

Dosage Form: chewable tablet, liquid

Active Ingredients: pseudoephedrine hydrochloride (HCl), chlorpheniramine maleate, acetaminophen, dextromethorphan hydrobromide

Warning: Do not use if carton is open, or if printed neck wrapper or printed foil inner seal is broken. Do not exceed recommended dosage. If nervousness, dizziness, or sleeplessness occur, discontinue use and consult a doctor. Do not take for pain for more than 5 days or for fever for more than 3 days, unless directed by a doctor. If pain or fever persists, gets worse, if new symptoms occur, or if redness or swelling is present, consult a doctor. These could be signs of a serious condition. If sore throat is severe, persists for more than 2 days, or is accompanied or followed by a fever, headache, rash, nausea or vomiting, consult a doctor promptly. A persistent cough may be a sign of a serious condition. If cough persists for more than 1 week, tends to recur, or is accompanied by a fever, rash or persistent headache, consult a doctor. Do not take this product for persistent or chronic cough such as occurs with asthma or if cough is accompanied by excessive phlegm (mucous) unless directed by a doctor. Do not give this product to children who have a breathing problem such as chronic bronchitis, or who have glaucoma, heart disease, high blood pressure, thyroid disease, or diabetes unless directed by a doctor. May cause excitability especially in children. May cause drowsiness; sedatives, and tranquilizers may increase its drowsiness effect. Do not give to children who are taking sedatives or tranquilizers without first consulting your doctor. Do not use with other products containing acetaminophen. DRUG INTER-ACTION PRECAUTION: Do not use this product if you are now taking a prescription monoamine oxidase inhibitor (MAOI) (certain drugs for depression, psychiatric or emotional conditions, or Parkinson's disease) or for 2 weeks after stopping the MAOI drug. If you are uncertain if your prescription drug contains an MAOI, consult a health professional before taking this product.

TYLENOL COLD MULTI-SYMPTOM
McNeil Consumer Products Company

Dosage Form: tablet, caplet

Active Ingredients: pseudoephedrine hydrochloride (HCl), chlorpheniramine maleate, acetaminophen, dextromethorphan hydrobromide

Warning: Do not use if carton is open, or if printed neck wrapper or printed foil inner seal is broken. If nervousness, dizziness, or sleeplessness occur, discontinue use and consult a doctor. Do not take for pain for more than 5 days or for fever for more than 3 days, unless directed by a doctor. If pain or fever persists, gets worse, if new symptoms occur, or if redness or swelling is present, consult a doctor. These could be signs of a serious condition. If sore throat is severe, persists for more than 2 days, or is accompanied or followed by a fever, headache, rash, nausea or vomiting, consult a doctor promptly. A persistent cough may be a sign of a serious condition. If cough persists for more than 1 week, tends to recur, or is accompanied by a fever, rash or persistent headache, consult a doctor. Do not take this product for persistent or

chronic cough such as occurs with asthma or if cough is accompanied by excessive phlegm (mucous) unless directed by a doctor. Do not give this product to children who have a breathing problem such as chronic bronchitis, or who have glaucoma, heart disease, high blood pressure, thyroid disease, or diabetes unless directed by a doctor. May cause excitability especially in children. May cause drowsiness; sedatives, and tranquilizers may increase its drowsiness effect. Do not give to children who are taking sedatives or tranquilizers without first consulting your doctor. Do not use with other products containing acetaminophen. DRUG INTER-ACTION PRECAUTION: Do not use this product if you are now taking a prescription monoamine oxidase inhibitor (MAOI) (certain drugs for depression, psychiatric or emotional conditions, or Parkinson's disease) or for 2 weeks after stopping the MAOI drug. If you are uncertain if your prescription drug contains an MAOI, consult a health professional before taking this product.

TYLENOL EXTRA STRENGTH
McNeil Consumer Products Company

Dosage Form: tablet, caplet

Active Ingredient: acetaminophen

Warning: Do not take for pain for more than 10 days or for fever for more than 3 days unless directed by a doctor. If pain or fever persists or gets worse, if new symptoms occur, or if redness or swelling is present, consult a doctor. These could be signs of serious illness. Do not use with any other products containing acetaminophen. If you generally consume 3 or more alcohol-containing drinks per day, you should consult your doctor for advice on when and how you should take this product and other pain relievers.

TYLENOL SINUS MAXIMUM STRENGTH
McNeil Consumer Products Company

Dosage Form: caplet, tablet, gelcap, geltab

Active Ingredients: pseudoephedrine hydrochloride (HCl), acetaminophen

Warning: Do not exceed recommended dosage because at higher dosages, nervousness, dizziness, or sleeplessness may occur. Do not take for pain for more than 7 days or for fever for more than 3 days unless directed by a doctor. If pain or fever persists, or gets worse, if new symptoms occur, or if redness or swelling is present, consult a doctor because these could be signs of a serious condition. Do not take this product if you have a breathing problem such as emphysema or chronic bronchitis, heart disease, high blood pressure, diabetes, thyroid disease, or if you have glaucoma or difficulty in urination due to enlargement of the prostate gland unless directed by a doctor. May cause excitability especially in children. May cause drowsiness; alcohol, sedatives, and tranquilizers may increase its drowsiness effect. Avoid alcoholic beverages while taking this product. Do not take this product if you are taking sedatives or tranquilizers without first consulting your doctor. Use caution while driving a motor vehicle or operating machinery. If you generally consume 3 or

more alcohol-containing drinks per day, you should consult your physician for advice on when and how you should take this product and other pain relievers. Do not use with other products containing acetaminophen. DRUG INTERACTION PRECAUTION: Do not use this product if you are now taking a prescription monoamine oxidase inhibitor (MAOI) (certain drugs for depression, psychiatric or emotional conditions, or Parkinson's disease) or for 2 weeks after stopping the MAOI drug. If you are uncertain if your prescription drug contains an MAOI, consult a health professional before taking this product.

U

UNISOM NIGHTTIME SLEEP AID
Pfizer Inc., Consumer Care Group

Dosage Form: tablet

Active Ingredient: doxylamine succinate

Warning: For adults only. Do not give to children under 12 years of age. If sleeplessness persists continuously for more than 2 weeks, consult a doctor. Insomnia may be a symptom of serious underlying medical illness. Do not take this product unless directed by a doctor, if you have breathing problems such as emphysema or chronic bronchitis, or if you have glaucoma, or difficulty in urination due to enlargement of the prostate gland. Avoid alcoholic beverages while taking this product. Do not take this product while taking any other drug, without consulting your doctor or pharmacist. This product contains an antihistamine and will cause drowsiness. It should be used only at bedtime.

UNISOM SLEEPGELS MAXIMUM STRENGTH
Pfizer Inc., Consumer Care Group

Dosage Form: softgel

Active Ingredient: diphenhydramine hydrochloride (HCl)

Warning: Do not give to children under 12 years of age. If sleeplessness persists continuously for more than 2 weeks, consult a doctor. Insomnia may be a symptom of serious underlying medical illness. Do not take this product unless directed by a doctor, if you have breathing problems such as emphysema or chronic bronchitis, or if you have glaucoma, or difficulty in urination due to enlargement of the prostate gland. Avoid alcoholic beverages while taking this product. Do not take this product if you are taking sedatives or tranquilizers without first consulting your doctor.

V

VASELINE INTENSIVE CARE EXTRA STRENGTH
Chesebrough-Pond's USA Company

Dosage Form: lotion

Active Ingredients: dimethicone

Warning: Avoid contact with eyes. If condition worsens or does not improve within 7 days, consult a doctor or pharmacist. Not to be applied over deep or puncture wounds, infections, or lacerations.

VASELINE LIP THERAPY
Chesebrough-Pond's USA Company

Dosage Form: stick, tube

Active Ingredients: white petrolatum

Warning: For external use only. Discontinue use if signs of irritation or rash occur. As with all personal care items, this product should be used by one individual only.

VASELINE LIP THERAPY ADVANCED FORMULA
Chesebrough-Pond's USA Company

Dosage Form: stick, tube

Active Ingredients: white petrolatum, ethylhexyl P-methoxycinnamate, oxybenzone

Warning: For external use only. Discontinue use if signs of irritation or rash occur. As with all personal care items, this product should be used by one individual only.

VICKS 44E PEDIATRIC COUGH & CHEST CONGESTION RELIEF
The Procter & Gamble Company

Dosage Form: liquid

Active Ingredients: guaifenesin, dextromethorphan hydrobromide

Warning: A persistent cough may be a sign of a serious condition. If cough persists for more than 1 week, tends to recur, or is accompanied by a fever, rash or persistent headache, consult a doctor. Do not take this product for persistent or chronic cough such as occurs with smoking, asthma, chronic bronchitis, or emphysema, or where cough is accompanied by excessive phlegm (mucous) unless directed by a doctor. DRUG INTERACTION PRECAUTION: Do not use this product if you are now taking a prescription monoamine oxidase inhibitor (MAOI) (certain drugs for depression, psychiatric or emotional conditions, or Parkinson's disease) or for 2 weeks after stopping the MAOI drug. If you are uncertain if your prescription drug contains an MAOI, consult a health professional before taking this product.

VICKS 44M COUGH, COLD & FLU RELIEF
The Procter & Gamble Company

Dosage Form: liquid

Active Ingredients: pseudoephedrine hydrochloride (HCl), chlorpheniramine maleate, acetaminophen, dextromethorphan hydrobromide

Warning: Do not exceed recommended dosage. If nervousness, dizziness, or sleeplessness occur, discontinue use and consult a doctor. Do not use this product for more than 7 days. If symptoms do not improve or are accompanied by a fever that lasts for more than 3 days, or if new symptoms occur, or if redness or swelling is present, consult a doctor. If sore throat is severe, persists for more than 2 days, or is accompanied or followed by a fever, headache, rash, nausea or vomiting, consult a doctor promptly. If cough persists for more than 1 week, tends to recur, or is accompanied by a rash, persistent headache, a fever that lasts for more than 3 days, or if new symptoms occur, consult a doctor. A persistent cough may be a sign of a serious condition. Do not take this product, if you have a breathing problem such as emphysema or chronic bronchitis, or if you have glaucoma, high blood pressure, heart disease, thyroid disease, diabetes or difficulty in urination due to the enlargement of the prostate gland, without first consulting a doctor. May cause excitability especially in children. May cause marked drowsiness; alcohol, sedatives, and tranquilizers may increase its drowsiness effect. Avoid alcoholic beverages while taking this product. Use caution while driving a motor vehicle or operating machinery. Do not use with other products containing acetaminophen. DRUG INTERACTION PRECAUTION: Do not take this product, without first consulting a doctor, if you take: sedatives, tranquilizers, a prescription monoamine oxidase inhibitor (MAOI) (certain drugs for depression, psychiatric or emotional conditions, or Parkinson's disease) or for 2 weeks after stopping the MAOI drug. If you are uncertain if your prescription drug contains an MAOI, consult a health professional before taking this product.

VICKS 44M PEDIATRIC COUGH & COLD RELIEF
The Procter & Gamble Company

Dosage Form: liquid

Active Ingredients: pseudoephedrine hydrochloride (HCl), chlorpheniramine maleate, dextromethorphan hydrobromide

Warning: Do not exceed recommended dosage because at higher dosages, nervousness, dizziness, or sleeplessness may occur. Do not take this product for more than 7 days. If symptoms do not improve or are accompanied by a fever, consult a doctor. A persistent cough may be a sign of a serious condition. If cough or other symptoms persist, do not improve within 7 days, tend to recur, or are accompanied by a fever, rash or persistent headache, consult a doctor. Do not take this product for persistent or chronic cough such as occurs with smoking,

asthma, chronic bronchitis, or emphysema, or if cough is accompanied by excessive phlegm (mucous) unless directed by a doctor. Do not take this product if you have a breathing problem such as emphysema or chronic bronchitis, or if you have heart disease, high blood pressure, diabetes, thyroid disease, glaucoma, or difficulty in urination due to enlargement of the prostate gland unless directed by a doctor. May cause excitability especially in children. May cause marked drowsiness; alcohol, sedatives, and tranquilizers may increase its drowsiness effect. Avoid alcoholic beverages while taking this product. Do not take this product while taking sedatives or tranquilizers without first consulting your doctor. Use caution while driving a motor vehicle or operating machinery. DRUG INTERACTION PRECAUTION: Do not use this product if you are now taking a prescription monoamine oxidase inhibitor (MAOI) (certain drugs for depression, psychiatric or emotional conditions, or Parkinson's disease) or for 2 weeks after stopping the MAOI drug. If you are uncertain if your prescription drug contains an MAOI, consult a health professional before taking this product.

VICKS CHLORASEPTIC SORE THROAT LOZENGES
The Procter & Gamble Company

Dosage Form: lozenge

Active Ingredients: benzocaine, menthol

Warning: If sore throat is severe, persists for more than 2 days, is accompanied or followed by a fever, headache, rash, swelling, nausea or vomiting, or is accompanied by difficulty in breathing, consult a doctor promptly. If sore throat symptoms do not improve within 7 days, or if irritation, pain, or redness persists or worsens, see your doctor promptly. Certain persons can develop allergic reactions to ingredients in this product. Do not use this product if you have a history of allergy to local anesthetics such as procaine, butacaine, benzocaine, or other "caine" anesthetics.

VICKS NYQUIL CHILDREN'S COLD/COUGH RELIEF
The Procter & Gamble Company

Dosage Form: liquid

Active Ingredients: pseudoephedrine hydrochloride (HCl), chlorpheniramine maleate, dextromethorphan hydrobromide

Warning: Do not exceed recommended dosage because at higher dosages, nervousness, dizziness, or sleeplessness may occur. Do not take this product for more than 7 days. If symptoms do not improve or are accompanied by a fever, consult a doctor. A persistent cough may be a sign of a serious condition. If cough or other symptoms persist, do not improve within 7 days, tend to recur, or are accompanied by a rash, persistent headache, or fever, consult a doctor. Do not take this product for persistent or chronic cough such as occurs with smoking, asthma, chronic bronchitis, or emphysema, or if cough is accompanied by excessive phlegm (mucous) unless directed by a doctor. Do not take this product if you have a breathing problem such as emphysema or chronic bronchitis, or if you have heart disease, high blood pressure, diabetes, thyroid disease, glaucoma, or difficulty in urination due to enlargement of the prostate gland unless directed by a doctor. May cause excitability especially in children. May cause marked drowsiness; alcohol, sedatives, and tranquilizers may increase its drowsiness effect. Avoid alcoholic beverages while taking this product. Do not take this product while taking sedatives or tranquilizers without first consulting your doctor. Use caution while driving a motor vehicle or operating machinery. DRUG INTERACTION PRECAUTION: Do not use this product if you are now taking a prescription monoamine oxidase inhibitor (MAOI) (certain drugs for depression, psychiatric or emotional conditions, or Parkinson's disease) or for 2 weeks after stopping the MAOI drug. If you are uncertain if your prescription drug contains an MAOI, consult a health professional before taking this product.

VICKS NYQUIL MULTI-SYMPTOM COLD/FLU RELIEF
The Procter & Gamble Company

Dosage Form: liquid, liqui cap, individual pack (powder)

Active Ingredients: pseudoephedrine hydrochloride (HCl), doxylamine succinate, acetaminophen, dextromethorphan hydrobromide

Warning: Do not exceed recommended dosage. If nervousness, dizziness, or sleeplessness occur, discontinue use and consult a doctor. Do not use this product for more than 7 days. If symptoms do not improve within 7 days or are accompanied by a fever that lasts for more than 3 days, or if new symptoms occur, or if redness or swelling is present, consult a doctor. If sore throat is severe, persists for more than 2 days, or is accompanied or followed by a fever, headache, rash, nausea or vomiting, consult a doctor promptly. If cough persists for more than 1 week, tends to recur, or is accompanied by a fever, rash or persistent headache, consult a doctor. A persistent cough may be a sign of a serious condition. Do not take this product for persistent or chronic cough such as occurs with smoking, asthma, emphysema, or if cough is accompanied by excessive phlegm (mucous) unless directed by a doctor. Do not take this product, if you have a breathing problem such as emphysema or chronic bronchitis, or if you have glaucoma, high blood pressure, heart disease, thyroid disease, diabetes or difficulty in urination due to the enlargement of the prostate gland, without first consulting a doctor. May cause excitability especially in children. May cause marked drowsiness; alcohol, sedatives, and tranquilizers may increase its drowsiness effect. Avoid alcoholic beverages while taking this product. Use caution while driving a motor vehicle or operating

machinery. Do not use with other products containing acetaminophen. DRUG INTERACTION PRECAUTION: Do not take this product, without first consulting a doctor, if you take: sedatives, tranquilizers, a prescription monoamine oxidase inhibitor (MAOI) (certain drugs for depression, psychiatric or emotional conditions, or Parkinson's disease) or for 2 weeks after stopping the MAOI drug. If you are uncertain if your prescription drug contains an MAOI, consult a health professional before taking this product.

VISINE ORIGINAL
Pfizer Inc., Consumer Care Group

Dosage Form: drops

Active Ingredient: tetrahydrozoline hydrochloride (HCl)

Warning: To avoid contamination of this product, do not touch tip of container to any surface. Replace cap after usage. If you experience eye pain, changes in vision, continued redness or irritation of the eye, or if the condition worsens or persists for more than 72 hours, discontinue use and consult a doctor. If you have glaucoma do not use this product except under the advice and supervision of a doctor. Overuse of this product may produce increased redness of the eye. If the solution changes color or becomes cloudy, do not use. Remove contact lenses before using this product. Before using with children under 6 years of age, consult your doctor.

WART-OFF WART REMOVER
Pfizer Inc., Consumer Care Group

Dosage Form: liquid

Active Ingredient: salicylic acid

Warning: For external use only. Do not use this product on irritated skin, on any area that is infected or reddened, if you are a diabetic, or if you have poor blood circulation. If discomfort persists, see your doctor. Do not use on moles, birthmarks, warts with hair growing from them, genital warts, or warts on the face or mucous membranes. If product gets in the eyes, flush with water for 15 minutes. Extremely flammable. Keep away from fire or flame. Avoid inhaling vapors.

X-SEB
Baker Cummins Dermatologicals

Dosage Form: shampoo

Active Ingredient: pyrithione zinc

Warning: For external use only. Avoid contact with the eyes. If contact occurs, rinse eyes thoroughly with water. If condition worsens or does not improve after regular use of this product as directed, consult a doctor. Do not use on children under 2 years of age, unless directed by a doctor.

X-SEB T PEARL
Baker Cummins Dermatologicals

Dosage Form: shampoo

Active Ingredient: coal tar solution

Warning: For external use only. Avoid contact with the eyes. If contact occurs, rinse eyes thoroughly with water. If condition worsens or does not improve after regular use of this product as directed, consult a doctor. Use caution in exposing skin to sunlight after applying this product. It may increase tendency to sunburn for up to 24 hours after application. Do not use for prolonged periods without consulting a doctor. Do not use this product with other forms of psoriasis therapy, such as ultraviolet radiation or prescription drugs, unless directed by a doctor. If condition covers large area of the body, consult your doctor before using this product. Do not use on children under 2 years of age, unless directed by a doctor. If undue irritation develops or increases, discontinue use and consult a doctor.

ZANTAC 75
Warner Wellcome Consumer

Dosage Form: tablet

Active Ingredient: ranitidine hydrochloride (HCl)

Warning: Do not take the maximum daily dose for more than 14 consecutive days, except under the advice and supervision of a doctor. If you have trouble swallowing or persistent abdominal pain, see a doctor promptly. You may have a serious condition that may need different treatment.

ZEASORB-AF
Stiefel Laboratories, Inc.

Dosage Form: powder

Active Ingredient: miconazole nitrate

Warning: For external use only. Do not use on children under 2 years of age except under the advice and supervision of a doctor. Avoid contact with the eyes. If irritation occurs or if there is no improvement within 4 weeks (for athlete's foot or ringworm) or within 2 weeks (for jock itch), discontinue use and consult a doctor or pharmacist.

ZILACTIN MEDICATED GEL
Zila Pharmaceuticals, Inc.

Dosage Form: gel

Active Ingredient: benzyl alcohol

Warning: Do not use in or near the eyes. In the event of accidental contact with the eyes, immediately flush with water. If pain or irritation persists with normal application, discontinue use and seek medical attention.

ZOSTRIX-HP HIGH POTENCY
GenDerm Corporation

Dosage Form: cream

Active Ingredient: capsaicin

Warning: For external use only. Use only as directed. Avoid contact with eyes and mucous membranes. If skin redness or irritation develops, if condition worsens, or does not improve within 7 days, or clears up and occurs again within a few days, discontinue use and consult a doctor. Do not apply to wounds, or to damaged, broken (open) or irritated skin. Do not bandage tightly. Do not use with a heating pad.

---

*When the pharmacists responded to the survey, Ciba Self-Medication, Inc. and Sandoz North American Consumer Pharmaceuticals were two independent manufacturers of over-the-counter products. On December 17, 1996, Ciba-Geigy Ltd. and Sandoz Ltd. received approval from the Federal Trade Commission to merge, forming Novartis. At this time Ciba Self-Medication and Sandoz Consumer Pharmaceuticals joined together to form Novartis Consumer Health.

Glossary

This section provides an alphabetical listing of the active ingredients found in the medications rated in this book and an explanation of their function.

acetaminophen
Pain reliever

activated charcoal
Relieves symptoms of gas and diarrhea

allantoin
Helps stimulate tissue repair and soothe dry skin

aloe
Plant extract used to treat dry skin and sunburn

alpha-galactosidase (enzyme)
Relieves gas by promoting the breakdown of complex sugars in the small intestine

alum
Antibacterial and antifungal agent

aluminum hydroxide
Antacid

amethicone
Silicone oil used to treat dry skin

aspirin
Pain reliever and anti-inflammatory agent

attapulgite
Used to treat diarrhea

**bacitracin
bacitracin zinc**
Antibiotic used in ointments

benzalkonium chloride
Antiseptic agent

benzocaine
Anesthetic applied to the skin

benzoin tincture compound
Protective ingredient that keeps tissue from becoming irritated, so that it can heal

benzoyl peroxide
Antibacterial agent that promotes the shedding of upper skin layers; used in medications to treat acne

benzyl alcohol
Anesthetic

bisacodyl
Laxative

bismuth subsalicylate
Antidiarrheal agent that reduces fluid secretion in the gastrointestinal tract. By coating the stomach, this agent relieves symptoms of heartburn, indigestion, and upset stomach

boric acid
Antibacterial and antifungal agent

brompheniramine maleate
Antihistamine

butoconazole nitrate
Antifungal agent used to treat vaginal yeast infections

calamine
Relieves pain and itching of skin rashes and allergies

calcium carbonate
Antacid; also used in pain relievers to decrease stomach upset

calcium polycarbophil
Laxative

camphor
Antiseptic

capsaicin
Topical analgesic used in creams to relieve muscle and joint pain

carbamide peroxide
Antibacterial agent with emollient effects; used to soften earwax and to treat minor oral irritation

carboxymethylcellulose sodium
Used in eyedrops as a lubricant

casanthranol
Laxative

cascara sagrada
Laxative

cetalkonium chloride
Topical antibacterial agent

cetyl alcohol
Moisturizer used in lip balms

chlorobutanol
Antimicrobial skin cleanser

chloroxylenol
Antibacterial agent

chlorpheniramine maleate
Antihistamine

cimetidine
Antiheartburn agent

clemastine fumarate
Antihistamine

clotrimazole
Antifungal agent

**coal tar
coal tar solution**
Used to treat skin and scalp conditions such as psoriasis and dandruff by reducing scale formation and increasing scale shedding

colloidal oatmeal
Used to soothe the skin

corn starch
Used in skin powders to prevent chafing, heat rash, and diaper rash

cyclizine hydrochloride (HCl)
Antihistamine used to treat nausea, vomiting, and motion sickness

dexbrompheniramine maleate
Antihistamine

dextran 70
Used to create artificial tears in eyedrops

dextromethorphan hydrobromide
Relieves coughs

dextromethorphan polistirex
Relieves coughs

dextrose
Decreases stomach and intestinal contractions to relieve symptoms of nausea and vomiting

dibasic sodium phosphate
Laxative

dimenhydrinate
Antihistamine used to relieve motion sickness

dimethicone
Silicone oil used to treat dry skin

diphenhydramine hydrochloride (HCl)
Antihistamine; also used in some sleeping pills

docusate calcium
Stool softener

docusate sodium
Stool softener

doxylamine succinate
Antihistamine. Also used in some sleeping pills

dried aluminum
Antacid

dyclonine hydrochloride (HCl)
Anesthetic used to relieve sore throats

ethylhexyl p-methoxycinnamate
Protects skin from ultraviolet radiation

eugenol
Clove oil; used as an antiseptic for the skin and as a soothing ingredient in dental medications

famotidine
Antiheartburn agent

glycerin
Hydrating agent used in many medicines, including eyedrops, skin lotions, and hemorrhoid treatments

guaifenesin
Aids in the elimination of bronchial secretions that contribute to nonproductive coughs

hydrocortisone
Mild steroid applied to the skin to relieve itching and swelling of many conditions

hydroxypropyl methylcellulose
Used to thicken eyedrops so they stay in your eyes

ibuprofen
Pain reliever and anti-inflammatory agent

isopropyl alcohol
Antiseptic and drying agent used externally

isopropyl myristate
Moisturizing agent used in lotions for dry skin and other topical products

ketoprofen
Pain reliever and anti-inflammatory agent

lanolin
Moisturizing agent

levulose
Decreases stomach and intestinal mobility to relieve symptoms of nausea and vomiting

lidocaine hydrochloride (HCl)
Anesthetic applied to the skin

loperamide hydrochloride (HCl)
Used to treat diarrhea

magaldrate
Antacid

magnesium carbonate
Antacid

magnesium hydroxide
Antacid

magnesium salicylate tetrahydrate
Pain reliever and anti-inflammatory agent

meclizine hydrochloride (HCl)
Antihistamine used to relieve motion sickness

menthol
Mild anesthetic used in creams and lotions to treat muscle and joint pain and in lozenges, for throat pain

methyl nicotinate
Topical analgesic used in creams to treat muscle and joint pain

methyl salicylate
Topical analgesic used in creams to treat muscle and joint pain

methylcellulose
Bulk-forming agent useful in the treatment of both constipation and diarrhea

miconazole nitrate
Antifungal medication

mineral oil
Moisturizing ingredient used in ointments and lotions

monobasic sodium phosphate
Laxative

naphazoline hydrochloride (HCl)
Used in eyedrops to relieve eye redness by constricting blood vessels

naproxen
Pain reliever and anti-inflammatory agent

neomycin
Antibiotic used in ointments

oxybenzone
Sun-blocking chemical used in sunscreens

oxymetazoline hydrochloride (HCl)
Reduces inflammation and congestion by constricting blood vessels; in eyedrops, used to relieve redness; in nasal sprays, used to relieve congestion

padimate O
Sun-blocking chemical used in sunscreens

permethrin
Kills parasites such as head lice

petrolatum
By itself, a moisturizer; in ointments, a base to hold medicine; taken internally, a laxative

phenindamine tartrate
Antihistamine

phenol
Disinfectant and anesthetic for the skin

phenolphthalein
Laxative

phenylephrine hydrochloride (HCl)
Reduces inflammation and congestion by constricting blood vessels

phenylpropanolamine hydrochloride (HCl)
Reduces inflammation and congestion by constricting blood vessels

phosphoric acid
Relieves nausea

piperonyl butoxide
Kills parasites such as head lice

polycarbophil
Absorbs water in the gastrointestinal tract; used in antidiarrheal medications or laxatives

polyethylene glycol
Used to thicken eyedrops so they stay in your eyes

polyethylene glycol 400
Treats eye irritation caused by allergies

polymyxin B sulfate
Antibiotic used on the skin

polyvinyl alcohol
Used as a soothing agent in artificial tears and eyedrops

povidone
Moisturizer used in eyedrops

povidone-iodine
Antibacterial and antifungal agent used externally

pramoxine hydrochloride (HCl)
Anesthetic applied to the skin

propylene glycol
Moisturizer used in lotions

pseudoephedrine hydrochloride (HCl)
Reduces inflammation and congestion by constricting blood vessels

pseudoephedrine sulfate
Reduces inflammation and congestion by constricting blood vessels

psyllium
psyllium hydrophilic mucilloid
Bulk-forming agent useful in the treatment of both constipation and diarrhea

pyrethrins
Kills parasites such as head lice

pyrethrum
pyrethrum extract
Kills parasites such as head lice

pyrithione zinc
Used to treat skin and scalp conditions such as psoriasis and dandruff by reducing scale formation and increasing scale shedding

ranitidine hydrochloride (HCl)
Antacid

salicylic acid
Mild antiseptic that causes skin to shed its upper layers; used in mild concentrations for acne medicine, and in strong concentrations to remove corns, calluses, and warts

salycin
Topical analgesic used in creams to relieve muscle and joint pain

selenium sulfide
Used to treat skin and scalp conditions such as psoriasis and dandruff by reducing scale formation and increasing scale shedding

senna concentrate
Laxative

sennosides
Laxative

simethicone
Relieves gas and indigestion

sodium benzoate
Antiseptic applied to the skin

sodium bicarbonate
Used to neutralize stomach acid

sodium chloride
Used to replace fluid in dry or irritated nasal passages

sulfur
Increases shedding of upper skin layers and has mild antifungal and antibacterial effects

tetrahydrozoline hydrochloride (HCl)
Reduces inflammation by constricting blood vessels; used in eyedrops to relieve redness

tolnaftate
Antifungal ingredient used to treat jock itch and athlete's foot

triclosan
Antibacterial and antifungal medication applied to the skin

triprolidine hydrochloride (HCl)
Antihistamine

trolamine salicylate
Used in lotions to treat muscle and joint pain

undecylenate
(as undecylenic witch hazel)
An astringent that soothes the skin

white petrolatum
See petrolatum

witch hazel
An astringent that soothes the skin

yellow phenolphthalein
See phenolphthalein

zinc chloride
Increases healing of oral lesions

zinc oxide
Possesses astringent, protective, and antiseptic effects; used to treat painful, itchy skin conditions such as diaper rash, dry skin and hemorrhoids

Writing
Elissa Keeler

Design and Production
Bernhardt Fudyma Design
Iris A. Brown
Nancy Caldwell
Kelly Holohan
Ignacio Rodriguez
Larry Wampler

Research
Burke Marketing Research
Mike Pietrangelo
Barb Jasper

Copy Editing
David Hall
Marge Wechsler

Special Thanks
To the American Pharmaceutical Association, especially
James Caro, Julian Graubart, Susan Kendall and
Ben Bluml.

To Iris Brown, Kelly Holohan and Ignacio Rodriguez for
their design input, and to Nancy Caldwell, Ignacio
Rodriguez and Larry Wampler for their assistance in the
production of this book.

To Marlyn Pollard for helping me coordinate the many
FedEx packages, phone conferences, and faxes.

To Bruce Canaday, Teresa Dunsworth, John Fudyma,
Paul Iverson, Leroy Knodel, and Stephen Rousch for
their knowledge, guidance, and time.

To my editors, Patricia Leasure and Rob Kaplan, for
guiding me through the process, and to their assistants,
Rob Amell and Jay Papasan for their support and
retrieval of information.

To Kathy D'Orazio for always finding my brother.

To Katherine Cowles, my agent, for making this book
a reality.

*Janice Fudyma received her B.F.A. from Syracuse
University and is a creative director and principal of the
Bernhardt Fudyma Design Group, which she cofounded
with her partner Craig Bernhardt in 1973.*

*Janice is responsible for the strategy, design, and creative
development of projects which range from corporate
identity to publishing and editorial design, general capa-
bilities/marketing materials, and corporate 'intra-net'
sites for such clients as American Express, Bear Stearns,
Nabisco Foods, Viacom, and many others.*

*Janice has received numerous awards for her work
from organizations such as the New York Art Director's
Club, The Los Angeles Art Director's Club, The
American Institute of Graphic Arts, and publications
such as* Communication Arts, Print *magazine, and* How
*magazine. In addition, the Library of Congress has
selected her firm's work for its permanent collection.*

Notes

Notes

Notes

Notes

Notes

Notes